the great thermo meal prep

COOKBOOK

Tracey Pattison is a qualified holistic health, wellbeing and
life coach with a 25-year career in cookbook publishing.
Her passion is encouraging people of all ages into the kitchen
in whichever way suits their lifestyle with a focus on
affordable, simply prepared and seasonal family food.

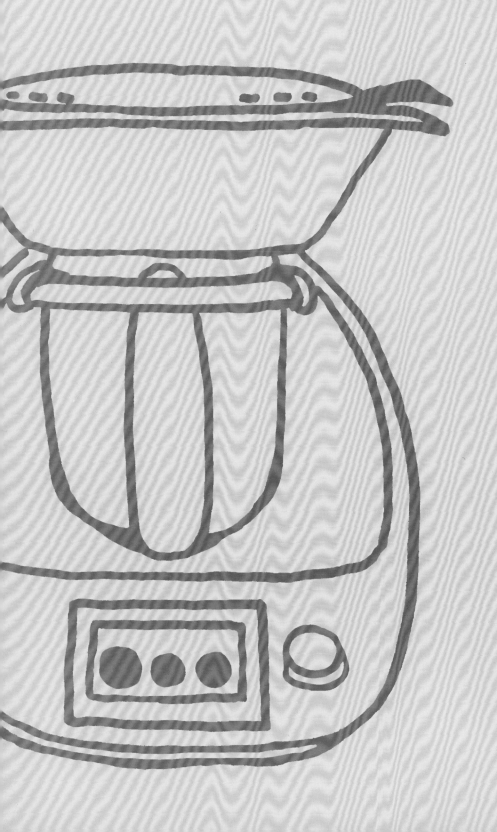

TRACEY
PATTISON

the great
thermo
meal prep
COOKBOOK

murdoch books

Sydney | London

contents

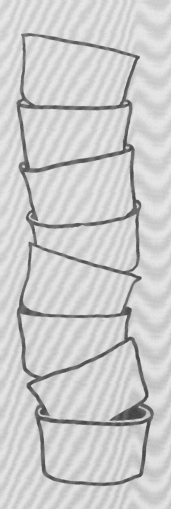

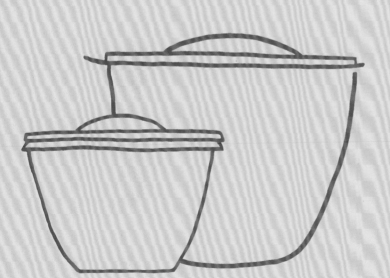

Welcome to The Great Thermo Meal Prep Cookbook!

There's nothing more satisfying than walking through the door at the end of a busy day and knowing you have a delicious meal just waiting to be quickly reheated or finished off in a flash – not one bought from the supermarket, but one you've lovingly made with your own hands, with no added nasties. This might be easier to achieve than you think if you are lucky enough to own a thermo appliance, and if you don't mind setting aside some time, weekly and monthly, to prep and cook a batch of meals to enjoy later.

If you're already in love with your thermo appliance – or if you've fallen out of love with it and perhaps been a bit harsh on yourself for not using it more often – then prepare yourself to reconnect, or connect even more deeply, with your beloved thermie.

Your machine will be like an extra pair of hands in the kitchen, doing much of the finicky work required in cooking, giving you the opportunity to make big-batch meals with ease, whip up mountains of baked goods, and fill your pantry, fridge and freezer with fresh spice blends, spice pastes, marinades, flavour boosters and flavour bases – which not only save you money, but taste oh-so-much-better than the store-bought alternatives.

In *The Great Thermo Meal Prep Cookbook*, I've got your weekdays, weeknights, weekends *and* special occasions all covered. There are mid-week meals, lunchbox fillers, weekend snacks for grazing, treats for surprise guests and transportable delights for taking to picnics, sports days and special events. This book is broken down into three easy sections, as described on the following pages.

IMPORTANT SAFETY NOTE

Please note that all recipes were written for, and tested in, a thermo appliance with a bowl capacity of 2.21 litres and steamer attachment capacity of 3.31 litres. Be sure to thoroughly read the disclaimer on page 240 for safety guidelines.

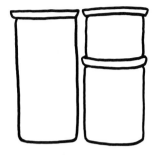

The great weeknight meals chapter

Here you'll find recipes for everyday flavour staples – such as dried spice blends and marinades, which will set your pantry and fridge up for a great week ahead – as well as dozens of recipes using them. Follow the 8-week menu plan, then spend a little time prepping on Sunday in order to stock your fridge with dinners for Monday, Tuesday and Wednesday – those first chaotic days of the week. As well as a prep list, each week's menu has its own shopping list, so all you have to do is take a photo of it on your phone, then head out to shop. Also in this chapter you'll find flavour boosters, which are designed to add to dishes to provide some extra fresh flavour and zing. I have included three uber-easy, five-ingredient recipes, which make use of each flavour booster.

The great batch-cook & freeze chapter

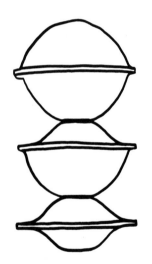

If you have the space, you can literally stack your freezer with a few weeks' – or even a few months' – worth of family meals, divided into ready-to-go portions. So that's what this chapter is all about – making big batches ahead of time, then freezing them. And next time you want to cook a curry, casserole or hotpot, you won't need to buy a paste or flavour base from the supermarket. In this chapter you'll find recipes to replace those store-bought versions. Better still, each recipe makes enough for several meals' worth, and you can simply divide the paste or flavour base into portions and refrigerate or freeze it until it's needed. Then, of course, I've also provided yummy recipes for curries, casseroles and hotpots that use the spice pastes and flavour bases. So grab your biggest wok, baking dish or stockpot and you're on your way.

The great make & bake ahead chapter

This chapter is all about creating big batches of scrumptious baked food that you can easily store. If you're after sweet or savoury dishes that you can transport easily and feed a crowd, then the Traybake & take section is for you. All you need are a couple of standard supermarket baking trays, and a little time to prep ahead, and you're set. Taking food to barbecues, picnics, sports days, birthday parties, school fetes or any other bring-a-plate affair has never been so easy, or tasty.

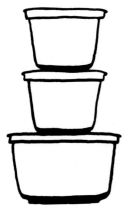

In the Bake & store section of this chapter you'll find simple grab-and-go snacks, as well as treats to bake ahead and store, then bring out of the pantry, fridge or freezer to enjoy anytime. These beauties will satisfy every tastebud requirement in your household as there's something for everyone.

And of course there are those lunchboxes that need to be filled, usually every day of the week, so the Lunchbox fillers section includes sweet and savoury options that are all freezer-friendly, and will fill tummies and keep little brains charged for the entire day. These recipes are not just for the kids – they are definitely enjoyed just as much by the adults!

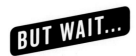

THERE IS EVEN MORE GREATNESS WAITING FOR YOU ONLINE!

Come and grab some extra free recipes and ideas, and we'll get to continue cooking together.

Use the link **traceypattison.com/great-thermo-cooks** and password MEALPREP to join the **Great Thermo Cooks** community. You will receive exclusive bonuses, such as extra recipes delivered to your inbox, video cooking tutorials, a great behind-the-scenes snapshot of how this book was created – as well as ME as your guide, in a closed Facebook group where we can share ideas and connect further as you use this fabulous book. I can't wait to welcome you there soon!

I'm so proud to be bringing you this cookbook, filled with recipes and ideas that utilise your thermo appliance, help to make your life easier and save you precious time. Happy cooking *The Great Thermo Meal Prep Cookbook* way!

With gratitude,
Tracey

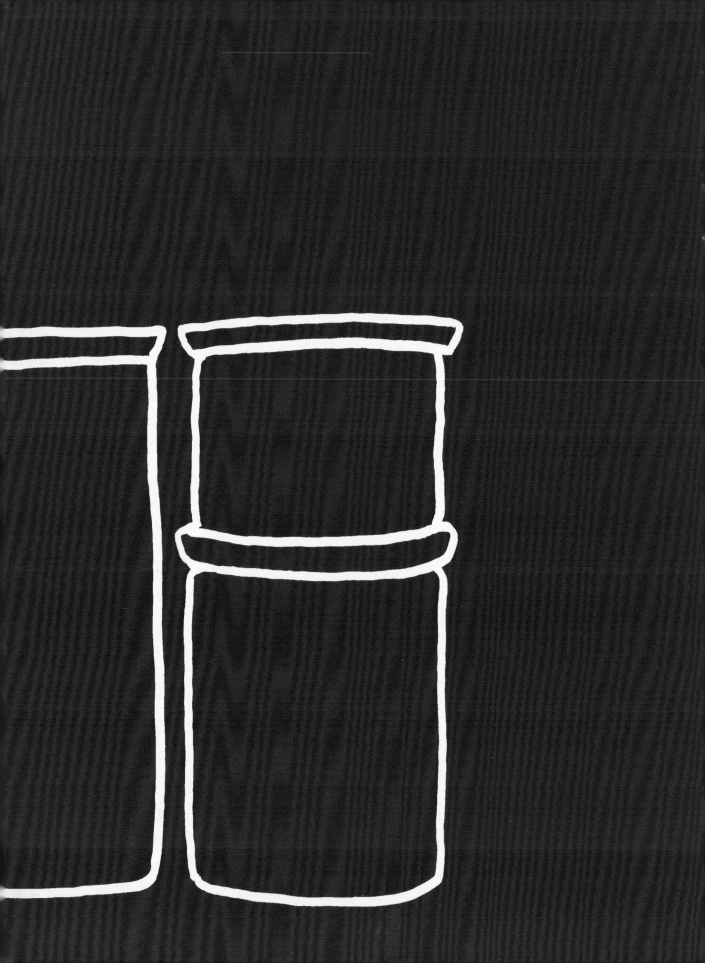

the great week-night meals chapter

everyday flavour staples

The starting point for getting prep-savvy with your thermo appliance is setting up your pantry and fridge with some go-to, family-friendly flavour staples, which you can have on-hand for those times during the week when all you have in the fridge are some random vegetables and proteins. So this is where we begin, with the building blocks that are the key to meal planning. The spice blends and marinades included in this chapter are easy to make ahead in large quantities, then you can just pull them out and use them to flavour a meal in no time at all. You'll see that with each of these flavour staples I've given you loads of inspiration with recipes and ideas on how you can use them in your everyday cooking. You'll see them featured not only in this section of the cookbook, but throughout later recipes, too – enjoy!

SPICE BLENDS

These spice blends can be stored in your pantry, fridge or freezer (depending on the quantity you decide to make) and will add life to any protein or vegetable before barbecuing, pan-frying, grilling (broiling) or baking. All the spice blends can be made ahead of time, and one quantity makes enough for a 6-serve meal. Add your chosen blend to your favourite protein (500–700 g/1 lb 2 oz–1 lb 9 oz) or vegetable combo (6 mixed chopped cups' worth) in a non-reactive dish, cover and keep chilled in the fridge for a minimum of 4 hours and maximum of up to 3 days.

STORAGE FOR SPICE BLENDS

1 full quantity
Store in an airtight container in a cool, dark pantry for up to 2 months.

2 full quantities
Store in an airtight container in the fridge for up to 3 months.

4 full quantities
Store in an airtight container in the freezer for up to 6 months. Just remove the quantity you need at any given time and store in the fridge in an airtight container until required.

MARINADES

The marinades can be stored in your fridge or freezer (depending on the quantity you decide to make) and are also designed to add flavour to any protein or vegetable before barbecuing, pan-frying, grilling (broiling) or baking. All the marinades can be made ahead of time, and one quantity makes enough for a 6-serve meal. Add your chosen marinade to your favourite protein (around 500–700 g/1 lb 2 oz–1 lb 9 oz) or vegetable combo (6 mixed chopped cups' worth) in a non-reactive dish, cover and keep chilled in the fridge for a minimum of 4 hours and maximum of up to 3 days.

STORAGE FOR MARINADES

1 full quantity
Store in an airtight container in the fridge for up to 1 week (fresh herbs will discolour slightly).

2 to 4 full quantities
Store in individual airtight containers in the freezer for up to 3 months. Just remove the quantity you need at any given time, defrost it in the fridge overnight and store the leftovers in the fridge in their airtight container until required.

Italian spice blend

makes approximately 45 g (1½ oz/¾ cup)
preparation 10 minutes

2 tablespoons dried marjoram
15 g (½ oz/¼ cup) dried basil
1 teaspoon dried chilli flakes
1 tablespoon dried rosemary
2 tablespoons dried oregano
2 tablespoons dried parsley
2 teaspoons dried thyme

Add all the ingredients to the mixer bowl, measuring cup in. Mill for 1 min/ speed 10 and repeat milling (scraping down the side of the bowl each time) until you have a fine powder. Transfer to an airtight container. Store in a cool, dark place for up to 3 months.

TRY THIS

Coat cubes of bread to make croutons

Add to drained tinned salmon and spread over toasted ciabatta

Pan-fry with sliced red onion and serve alongside steak

Cook with extra virgin olive oil and sliced garlic and toss through cooked spaghetti

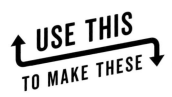

USE THIS TO MAKE THESE

Marinated mushrooms

In a large, clean airtight jar, combine 700 g (1 lb 9 oz) halved baby button mushrooms, 2 tablespoons of the spice blend, 1 teaspoon caster (superfine) sugar, 250 ml (9 oz/1 cup) red wine vinegar, 1 tablespoon dill leaves, 2 tablespoons finely chopped flat-leaf (Italian) parsley and 125 ml (4 fl oz/½ cup) extra virgin olive oil, making sure the mushrooms are completely submerged in the liquid. Close the jar and marinate at room temperature for 2 hours, shaking the jar occasionally. Chill for up to 1 week. Serve as part of a mezze, or as a snack with cheese and crackers.

Barbecued ratatouille

Combine 125 ml (4 fl oz/½ cup) olive oil; 60 ml (2 fl oz/¼ cup) red wine vinegar; 15 g (½ oz/¼ cup) of the spice blend; 1 large eggplant (aubergine), chopped; 6 roma (plum) tomatoes, quartered; 2 red onions, cut into wedges; 6 zucchini (courgettes), thickly sliced; 180 g (6½ oz/1 cup) pitted kalamata olives; 210 g (7½ oz/1 cup) semi-dried (sun-blushed) tomatoes in oil; 6 quartered garlic cloves and 60 g (2¼ oz/2 cups) basil leaves. Marinate for 2 hours. Cook on a barbecue flatplate on high for 8–10 minutes, or until just tender and starting to caramelise. Serve hot or store in an airtight container in the fridge for up to 1 week. Serve with any barbecued protein and a salad.

Easy pasta sauce

Combine 80 ml (2½ fl oz/⅓ cup) extra virgin olive oil, 3 crushed garlic cloves, 1.6 kg (3 lb 8 oz) tinned crushed tomatoes and 2 tablespoons of the spice blend in a large, deep frying pan over low heat. Simmer gently, stirring occasionally, for 25–30 minutes or until the sauce is rich and thick. Stir in 15 g (½ oz/½ cup) torn basil leaves. Serve hot or store in an airtight container in the fridge for up to 4 days.

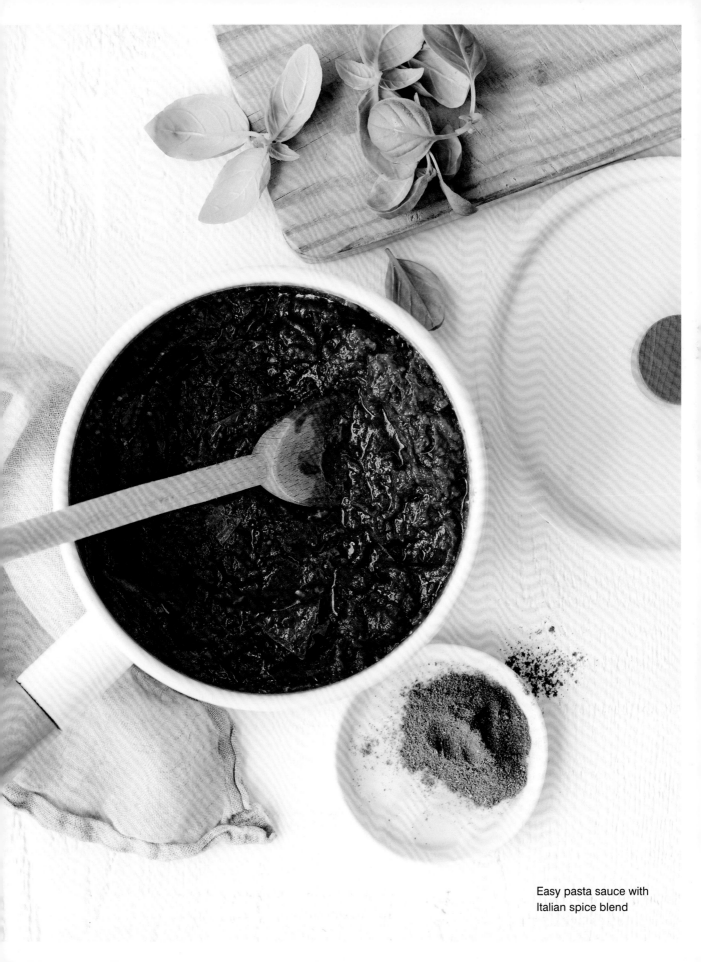

Easy pasta sauce with
Italian spice blend

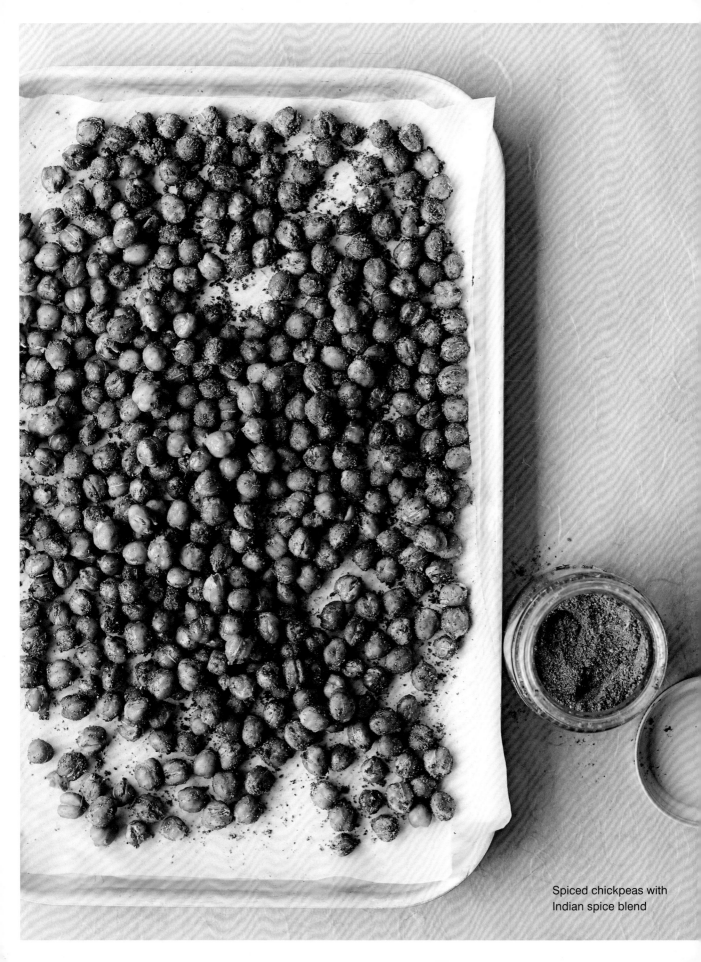

Spiced chickpeas with
Indian spice blend

Indian spice blend

makes approximately 70 g (2½ oz/¾ cup)
preparation 10 minutes

1 tablespoon black peppercorns
2 tablespoons caraway seeds
2 tablespoons fennel seeds
2 teaspoons cardamom pods
3 cinnamon sticks, broken into 3
2 teaspoons whole cloves

Add all the ingredients to the mixer bowl, measuring cup in. Mill for 1 min/speed 10 and repeat milling (scraping down the side of the bowl each time) until you have a fine powder. Transfer to an airtight container. Store in a cool, dark place for up to 3 months.

TRY THIS

Sprinkle over salmon fillets before grilling (broiling)

Add to yoghurt for marinades

Sprinkle over sliced cucumber for adding to lunch wraps

Sprinkle over flat breads before grilling

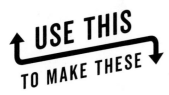

Spiced chickpeas

Drain and rinse 1.2 kg (2 lb 12 oz) tinned chickpeas, then toss with 2 tablespoons of the spice blend. Roast on a baking paper–lined baking tray in a preheated 220°C (425°F) oven (200°C/400°F fan-forced) for 25–30 minutes or until crisp and dark golden. Cool on the tray. Serve as a snack.

Lentil and cauliflower soup

Cook 2 tablespoons of the spice blend with 1 chopped onion, 410 g (14½ oz/2 cups) split red lentils, 600 g (1 lb 5 oz) cauliflower florets and 1.5 litres (52 fl oz/ 6 cups) vegetable stock in a large saucepan over medium–low heat for 20–25 minutes, or until the lentils are very soft and the cauliflower is falling apart. Serve.

Simple pilaf

Cook 2 tablespoons of the spice blend with 2 finely chopped red onions and 50 g (1¾ oz) butter in a large saucepan over medium heat for 10 minutes until very soft and dark golden. Add 400 g (14 oz/2 cups) white basmati rice, stir for 1 minute to coat the rice well in the mixture, then add 1 litre (35 fl oz/4 cups) vegetable stock. Immediately reduce the heat to the lowest possible setting, cover with a lid and leave to cook, untouched, for 18–20 minutes or until the rice is cooked and the stock has been absorbed. Remove the pan from the heat and stand for 3 minutes. Use a fork to fluff up the rice and separate the grains. Serve as a side with Indian dishes.

Mexican spice blend

makes approximately 70 g (2½ oz/⅔ cup)
preparation 10 minutes

2 teaspoons black peppercorns
2 tablespoons cumin seeds
1 tablespoon dried chilli flakes
1 tablespoon dried oregano
1 tablespoon garlic powder
2 tablespoons sweet paprika

1 Add the peppercorns and cumin seeds to the mixer bowl, measuring cup in. Mill for 1 min/speed 10. Scrape down the side of the bowl.

2 Add the chilli flakes and oregano, measuring cup in. Mill for 1 min/speed 10. Scrape down the side of the bowl.

3 Add the garlic powder and paprika, measuring cup in. Mill for 1 min/speed 10 until you have a fine powder. Repeat if needed. Transfer to an airtight container. Store in a cool, dark place for up to 3 months.

TRY THIS

Add a little to tomato juice before drinking

Toss through cauliflower florets before roasting

Toss through drained and rinsed tinned red kidney beans, then use to fill whole baked potatoes

Sprinkle over mountain breads before roasting to make 'dipper' shards

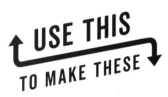

Mexican wedges

Cut 1.5 kg (3 lb 5 oz) sweet potatoes into wedges and place in a large, heavy-based baking dish. Add 80 ml (2½ fl oz/⅓ cup) avocado oil and 30 g (1 oz/¼ cup) of the spice blend, tossing to coat the potatoes well in the mixture. Roast in a preheated 220°C (425°F) oven (200°C/400°F fan-forced) for 50 minutes, turning occasionally, or until cooked and crisp. Serve hot.

Spicy beef stew

In a saucepan over high heat, brown 700 g (1 lb 9 oz) minced (ground) beef, 2 chopped red onions, 30 g (1 oz/¼ cup) of the spice blend and 60 ml (2 fl oz/¼ cup) avocado oil for 15 minutes or until golden. Reduce the heat to low and add 800 g (1 lb 12 oz) drained and rinsed tinned red kidney beans, 800 g (1 lb 12 oz) tinned crushed tomatoes, 800 g (1 lb 12 oz) quartered baby potatoes and 500 ml (17 fl oz/2 cups) beef stock. Simmer gently, partially covered and stirring occasionally, for 20–25 minutes or until cooked and the sauce reduces and thickens. Serve with rice.

Loaded avo dip

Smash together 4 avocados, 2 tablespoons of the spice blend, the kernels from 2 corn cobs, 1 finely chopped green capsicum (pepper), 250 g (9 oz) quartered cherry tomatoes, 4 thinly sliced spring onions (scallions), the finely grated zest and juice of 1 large lemon and ¼ teaspoon dried chilli flakes. Serve with fresh vegetable sticks.

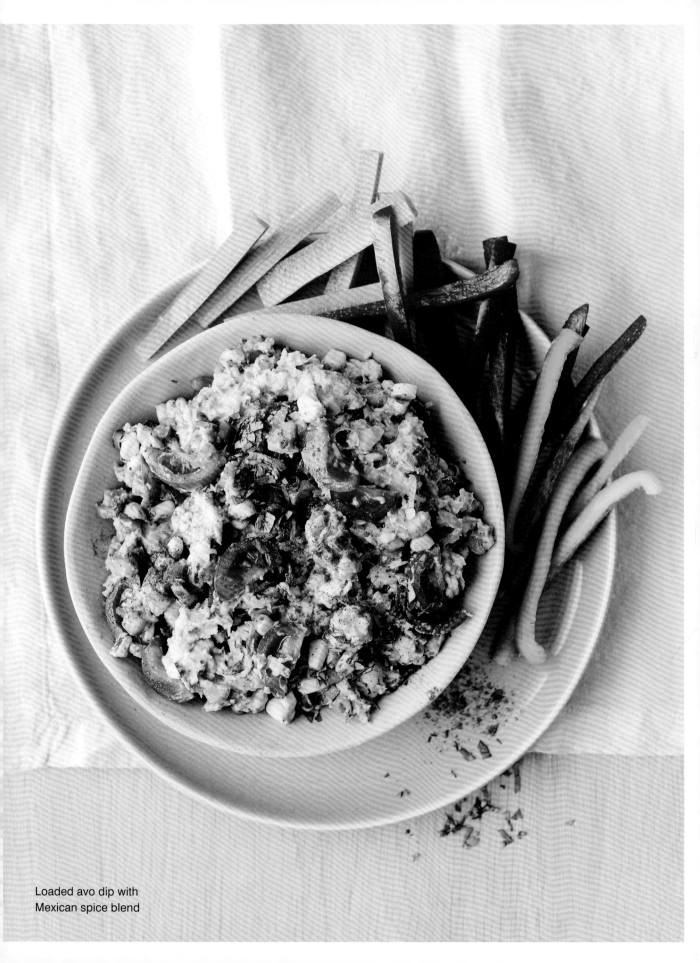

Loaded avo dip with
Mexican spice blend

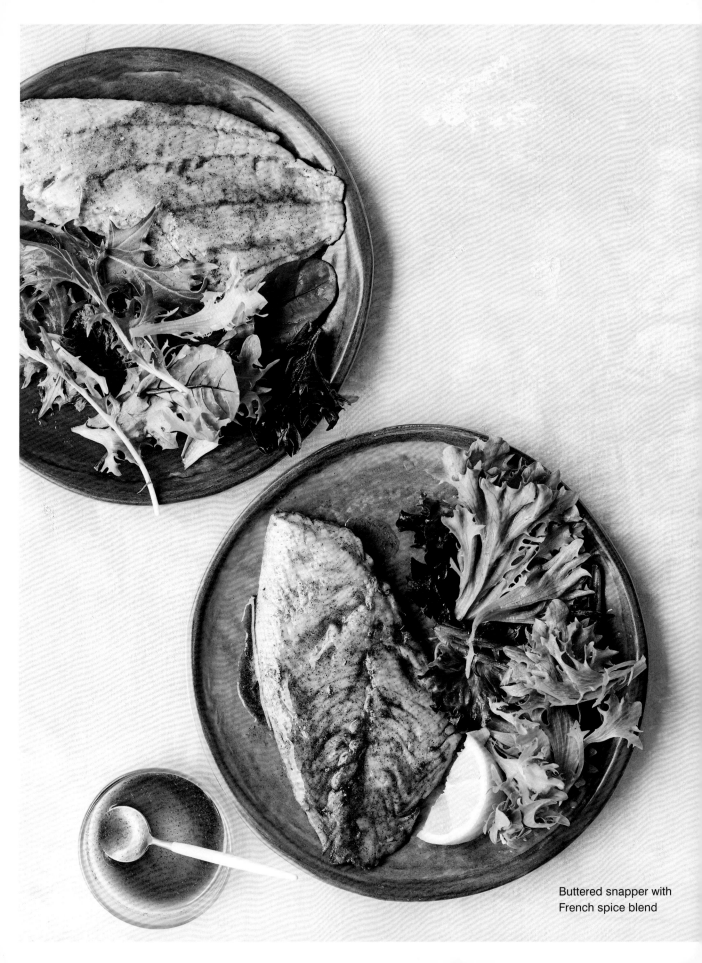

Buttered snapper with
French spice blend

French spice blend

makes approximately 35 g (1¼ oz/½ cup)
preparation 10 minutes

2 tablespoons dried thyme
1 tablespoon dried rosemary
1 tablespoon dried basil
2 tablespoons dried parsley
2 teaspoons dried oregano
2 tablespoons dried tarragon
2 teaspoons dried marjoram

Add all the ingredients to the mixer bowl, measuring cup in. Mill for 1 min/speed 10 and repeat milling (scraping down the side of the bowl each time) until you have a fine powder. Transfer to an airtight container. Store in a cool, dark place for up to 3 months.

TRY THIS

Add to white wine vinegar for a no-oil dressing

Sprinkle over any vegetable soup

Sprinkle over zucchini (courgette) halves before barbecuing

Rub over skinless chicken breast fillets before cooking in a chargrill pan

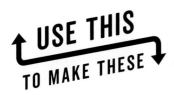

Buttered snapper

Lightly dust 6 x 200 g (7 oz) skinless, boneless snapper fillets in flour. Working with one fillet at a time, melt 25 g (1 oz) butter and 2 teaspoons olive oil in a large non-stick frying pan over medium–high heat. Add 2 teaspoons of the spice blend, then 1 snapper fillet. Cook for 4 minutes on one side, carefully turn, then cook for 4–5 minutes on the other side. Transfer the fish to a plate and pour over the butter mixture from the pan. Serve with lemon wedges and a mixed leaf salad.

Braised fennel and leek

Place 2 thinly sliced leeks, 6 thinly sliced baby fennel bulbs, 2 crushed garlic cloves, 15 g (½ oz/¼ cup) of the spice blend and 50 g (1¾ oz) butter in a large saucepan over medium–low heat. Cook, covered and stirring occasionally, for 20 minutes or until very soft. Serve with the pan-fried protein of your choice and a salad.

Lemon drumsticks

Combine 12 large chicken drumsticks with the skin scored, 15 g (½ oz/¼ cup) of the spice blend, 2 sliced lemons, 2 thickly sliced red onions, 4 sliced zucchini (courgettes) and 125 ml (4 fl oz/ ½ cup) extra virgin olive oil in a large baking dish, tossing together well and making sure everything is evenly coated in the mixture. Bake in a preheated 200°C (400°F) oven (180°C/350°F fan-forced) for 55–60 minutes, turning occasionally, or until the chicken is cooked and golden. Serve with a mixed salad.

All-purpose spice blend

makes approximately 70 g (2½ oz/¾ cup)
preparation 10 minutes

1 tablespoon black peppercorns
2 tablespoons celery seeds
1 tablespoon dried basil
2 tablespoons dried onion flakes
2 tablespoons garlic powder
2 tablespoons sweet paprika

1 Add the peppercorns and celery seeds to the mixer bowl, measuring cup in. Mill for 1 min/speed 10. Scrape down the side of the bowl.

2 Add the basil and onion flakes, measuring cup in. Mill for 1 min/speed 10. Scrape down the side of the bowl.

3 Add the garlic powder and paprika, measuring cup in. Mill for 1 min/speed 10 until you have a fine powder. Repeat if needed. Transfer to an airtight container. Store in a cool, dark place for up to 3 months.

TRY THIS

Sprinkle over onions before pan-frying

Sprinkle over sweet potato fries before roasting

Add to any meatball mixture

Use as a flavour base for savoury mince

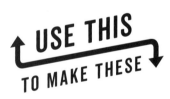

USE THIS TO MAKE THESE

Grilled tomatoes

Halve 6 vine-ripened tomatoes and place them, cut side up, on a foil-lined baking tray. Sprinkle evenly with 1 tablespoon of the spice blend, then drizzle with 1 tablespoon avocado oil. Cook under a grill (broiler) on high, for 8–10 minutes or until the tomatoes are soft and starting to split, and the tops are golden. Serve with eggs for breakfast or over toasted bread for brunch.

Barbecue lamb rack

Rub 1 tablespoon of the spice blend over 2 six-point lamb cutlet racks. Cook on a preheated barbecue on medium–high for 8–10 minutes, turning occasionally, for medium, or cook to your liking. Slice and serve with your favourite potato salad.

Roast potatoes

In a large roasting tin, toss together 500 g (1 lb 2 oz) peeled and chopped all-purpose potatoes, 60 ml (2 fl oz/¼ cup) macadamia oil and 1 tablespoon of the spice blend. Roast in a preheated 200°C (400°F) oven (180°C/350°F fan-forced) for 45–50 minutes, turning occasionally, or until cooked and crisp. Serve alongside your favourite barbecued, grilled (broiled) or pan-fried protein, with a salad or extra steamed vegies.

Thai spice blend

makes approximately 95 g (3¼ oz/1 cup)
preparation 10 minutes

2 tablespoons cumin seeds
2 tablespoons coriander seeds
3 teaspoons dried basil
1 tablespoon dried onion flakes
2 teaspoons dried chilli flakes
1 tablespoon garlic powder
2 tablespoons ground lemongrass
1 tablespoon ground ginger
2 teaspoons ground turmeric

1 Add the cumin and coriander seeds to the mixer bowl, measuring cup in. Mill for 1 min/speed 10. Scrape down the side of the bowl.

2 Add the basil, onion and chilli flakes, measuring cup in. Mill for 1 min/speed 10. Scrape down the side of the bowl.

3 Add the remaining ingredients, measuring cup in. Mill for 1 min/speed 10 until you have a fine powder. Repeat if needed. Transfer to an airtight container. Store in a cool, dark place for up to 3 months.

TRY THIS

Use as a flavour base for soup

Add to drained tinned tuna and use as a cracker topping

Stir through steamed jasmine rice before serving

Sprinkle over steamed sugar snap peas

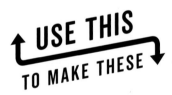

USE THIS TO MAKE THESE

Best-ever dressing

In a screw-top jar, place 2 tablespoons of the spice blend, 2 tablespoons caster (superfine) sugar, 2 tablespoons lime juice, 1 tablespoon Thai fish sauce, 2 tablespoons macadamia oil and 1 finely chopped long red chilli. Screw the lid on tightly and shake the jar until the sugar dissolves. Use for anything that requires a dressing.

Thai chicken rolls

Toss 500 g (1 lb 2 oz) shredded barbecued chicken meat with 2 tablespoons of the spice blend. Spread 6 crunchy long bread rolls each with 1 tablespoon mayonnaise, then top evenly with 120 g (4¼ oz/2 cups) shredded iceberg lettuce, then 2 Lebanese (short) cucumbers cut into ribbon slices with a peeler, and finally the chicken mixture.

Thai calamari

Toss 2 tablespoons of the spice blend with 700 g (1 lb 9 oz) cleaned and scored baby squid hoods before cooking on a preheated barbecue chargrill plate on high for 5–6 minutes. Remove the calamari and toss it with watercress leaves. Serve with lime wedges.

Chinese spice blend

makes approximately 50 g (1¾ oz/⅔ cup)
preparation 10 minutes

2 cinnamon sticks, broken into 3
2 whole star anise
2 teaspoons whole cloves
2 tablespoons fennel seeds
10 g (¼ oz/¼ cup) szechuan peppercorns

Add all the ingredients to the mixer bowl, measuring cup in. Mill for
1 min/speed 10 and repeat milling (scraping down the side of the bowl
each time) until you have a fine powder. Transfer to an airtight container.
Store in a cool, dark place for up to 3 months.

TRY THIS

Sprinkle over crispy Asian
omelettes

**Sprinkle over mixed
mushrooms before chargrilling**

Mix with hoisin for a quick
dipping sauce for spring rolls

Add to a crispy noodle salad

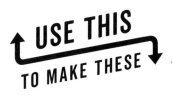

USE THIS TO MAKE THESE

Barbecue pork

Roll 700 g (1 lb 9 oz) trimmed
pork fillet in 20 g (¾ oz/¼ cup)
of the spice blend. Cook on a
preheated barbecue chargrill plate
on high for 10–12 minutes until
cooked and golden. Serve sliced
with steamed Asian greens and
soy sauce drizzled over.

Chicken lettuce cups

In a large wok over high heat,
stir-fry 600 g (1 lb 5 oz) minced
(ground) chicken, 2 tablespoons
macadamia oil, 2 tablespoons of
the spice blend and 225 g (8 oz)
tinned water chestnuts (drained
and rinsed, then finely chopped)
for 10 minutes or until cooked.
Remove from the heat, then toss
through 4 thinly sliced spring
onions (scallions) before spooning
the mixture into 12 iceberg lettuce
cups. Drizzle each with ½ teaspoon
oyster sauce. Serve.

Crispy tofu

Cut 700 g (1 lb 9 oz) firm tofu into
2 cm (¾ inch) pieces and pat dry
with paper towel. Coat in 20 g
(¾ oz/¼ cup) of the spice blend,
then stir-fry in batches in hot
sesame oil for 2 minutes or until
crispy. Serve tossed through
250 g (9 oz) soaked and drained
rice vermicelli, 30 g (1 oz/1 cup)
coriander (cilantro) leaves and
finally drizzle over the juice of
1 lemon.

Moroccan spice blend

makes approximately 90 g (3¼ oz/1 cup)
preparation 10 minutes

2 teaspoons black
  peppercorns
2 tablespoons coriander
  seeds
2 tablespoons cumin seeds
3 teaspoons dried onion flakes

3 teaspoons dried rosemary
2 teaspoons dried chilli flakes
3 teaspoons garlic powder
1 tablespoon sweet paprika
1 tablespoon ground turmeric
2 teaspoons ground ginger

TRY THIS

Sprinkle over beef topside
before roasting

**Use as a flavour base for
sweet potato soup**

Add to shredded barbecued
chicken and mayo for a simple
sandwich filler

**Add to peeled raw prawns
(shrimp) before chargrilling**

1 Add the peppercorns and the coriander and cumin seeds to the mixer
   bowl, measuring cup in. Mill for 1 min/speed 10. Scrape down the side
   of the bowl. Add the onion flakes, rosemary and chilli flakes, measuring
   cup in. Mill for 1 min/speed 10. Scrape down the side of the bowl.

2 Add the remaining ingredients, measuring cup in. Mill for 1 min/
   speed 10 until you have a fine powder. Repeat if needed. Transfer to
   an airtight container. Store in a cool, dark place for up to 3 months.

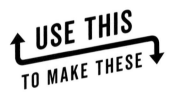

Moroccan rice

In a pan over medium heat add
4 tablespoons olive oil, 2 chopped
onions, 45 g (1½ oz/½ cup) of the
spice blend and 60 g (2¼ oz/¼ cup)
tomato paste (concentrated purée).
Cook until soft. Add 300 g (10½ oz/
2½ cups) long-grain white rice and
1 litre (35 fl oz/4 cups) vegetable
stock. Stir, then reduce the heat
to very low. Cook, covered, for
18–20 minutes or until tender and
the stock is absorbed. Remove
from the heat. Add 130 g (4½ oz/
1 cup) peas. Stand, covered, for
5 minutes. Use a fork to fluff and
separate the rice. Serve sprinkled
with flat-leaf (Italian) parsley, lemon
wedges and pan-fried chicken.

Pickled onions

Using a mandoline, very thinly
slice 3 red onions. Place in a
glass bowl. Add 2 tablespoons
of the spice blend, 1 teaspoon
caster (superfine) sugar and 250 ml
(9 fl oz/1 cup) white wine vinegar.
Toss well to combine and coat
everything in the mixture. Stand,
covered, for at least 2 hours,
turning occasionally or until the
onions have softened. Serve with
grilled meats, chicken or seafood.

Easy tagine

In a non-stick frying pan over
medium heat, add 80 ml (2½ fl oz/
⅓ cup) olive oil, 3 chopped garlic
cloves, 20 g (¾ oz/¼ cup) of the
spice blend and 2 chopped red
onions. Cook for 5 minutes until
softened. Add 700 g (1 lb 9 oz)
chopped skinless chicken breast
fillets. Cook for 10 minutes or until
light golden. Add 2 chopped
carrots; 2 chopped zucchini
(courgettes); 4 roma (plum)
tomatoes, quartered lengthways;
and 250 ml (9 fl oz/1 cup) chicken
stock. Reduce to low, then simmer,
uncovered, for 20 minutes or until
reduced by half. Serve with rice.

Thai spiced marinade

makes approximately 230 g (8½ oz/1¾ cups)
preparation 10 minutes

15 g (½ oz/½ cup) Thai basil leaves
2 tablespoons Thai spice blend (page 23)
3 teaspoons fish sauce
zest and juice of 4 large limes
2 teaspoons white sugar
125 ml (4 fl oz/½ cup) macadamia oil

1   Add the Thai basil to the mixer bowl, measuring cup in. Chop for
    3 sec/speed 7. Scrape down the side of the bowl.

2   Add the remaining ingredients to the mixer bowl, measuring cup in.
    Combine for 5 sec/speed 5.

TRY THIS

Use as a dressing for salads

Toss through hot, cooked noodles before serving

Use to marinate tofu before pan-frying

Toss through Asian greens before stir-frying

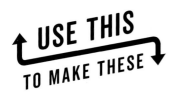

USE THIS TO MAKE THESE

Barramundi parcels

Place 6 x 200 g (7 oz) skinless, boneless barramundi (or other thick-flake white fish) portions onto doubled squares of foil. Top evenly with 300 g (10½ oz) trimmed snow peas (mangetout); 1 thinly sliced large red onion and 250 g (9 oz) baby corn, halved lengthways. Spoon over the marinade, then wrap the parcels up tightly. Cook directly on the shelves of a preheated 220°C (425°F) oven (200°C/400°F fan-forced) for 20 minutes until cooked. Serve.

Marinated beans

Steam 400 g (14 oz) trimmed baby green beans, 400 g (14 oz) trimmed snow peas (mangetout), 400 g (14 oz) trimmed sugar snap peas and 170 g (6 oz/1 cup) shelled edamame for 2 minutes until just tender. Combine the vegetables with the marinade and stand for 5 minutes, tossing occasionally. Serve with your favourite grilled seafood or chicken.

Chicken tenders

Combine 700 g (1 lb 9 oz) chicken tenderloins and the marinade in a flat ovenproof dish, turning to coat the chicken well in the mixture. Cover and chill for at least 2 hours or overnight. Remove the dish from the fridge and leave to stand at room temperature for 10 minutes. Sprinkle the top of the chicken tenderloins with 90 g (3 oz/1½ cups) Japanese (panko) breadcrumbs and 40 g (1½ oz/½ cup) finely chopped cashews. Bake in a preheated 220°C (425°F) oven (200°C/400°F fan-forced) for 25–30 minutes or until the chicken is cooked, golden and crisp. Serve with salad and lemon wedges.

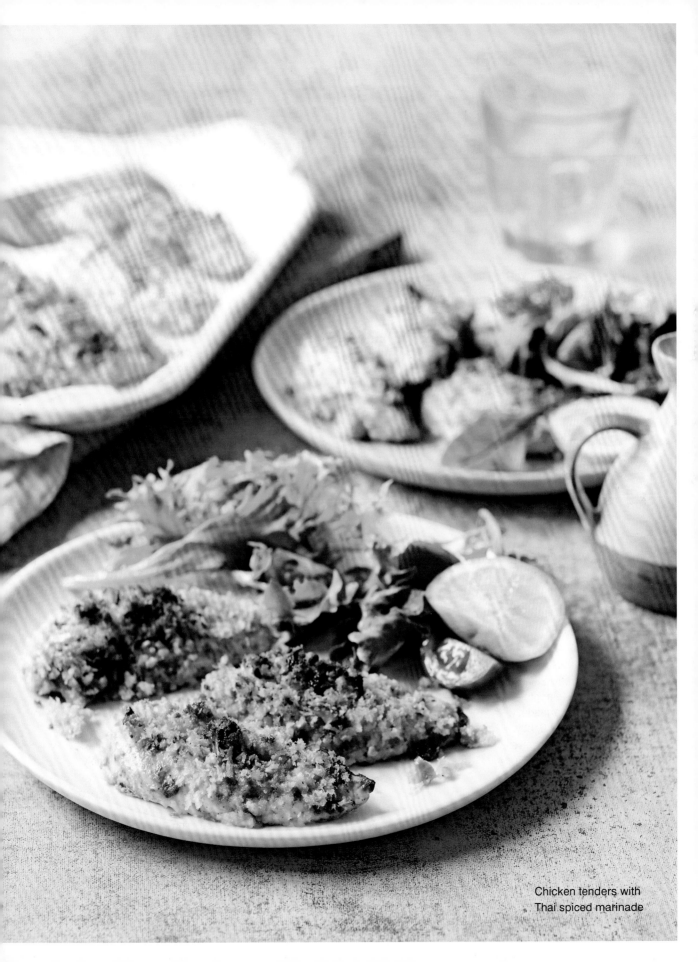

Chicken tenders with
Thai spiced marinade

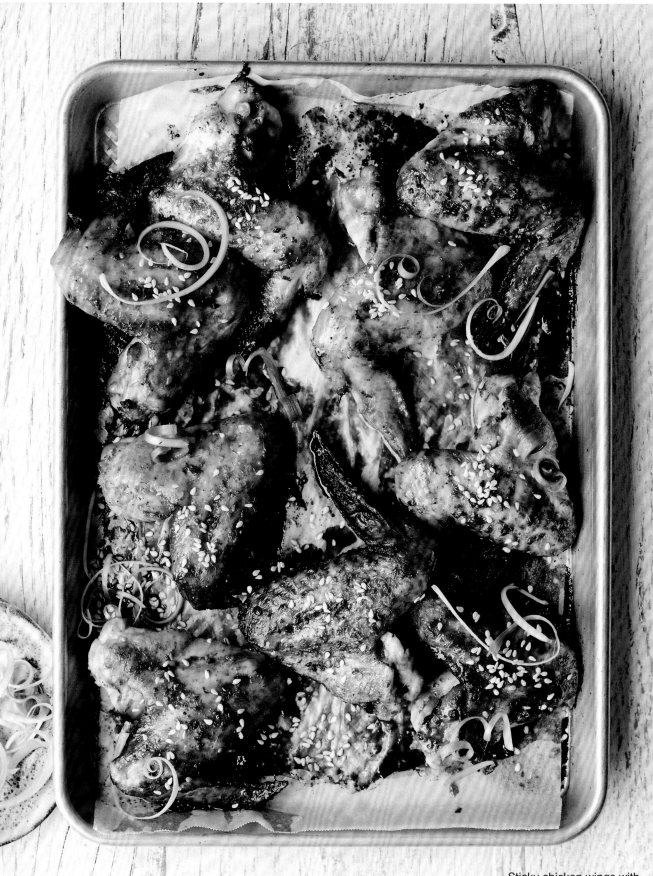

Sticky chicken wings with
sweet soy marinade

Sweet soy marinade

makes approximately 290 g (10¼ oz/1¾ cups)
preparation 10 minutes

2 tablespoons Chinese spice paste (page 128)
80 ml (2½ fl oz/⅓ cup) pure maple syrup
125 ml (4 fl oz/½ cup) soy sauce
1 tablespoon sesame seeds
125 ml (4 fl oz/½ cup) macadamia oil

Add all the ingredients to the mixer bowl, measuring cup in. Combine for 5 sec/speed 5.

TRY THIS

Sprinkle over salmon portions before barbecuing

Drizzle over stir-fried Asian greens

Drizzle over chargrilled white fish fillets

Use to marinate beef strips before stir-frying

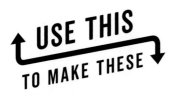

Sticky chicken wings

Combine the marinade and 2 kg (4 lb 8 oz) small chicken wings in a large bowl. Cover and chill for at least 2 hours or overnight to marinate. Transfer to two large baking paper–lined baking trays and cook in a preheated 200°C (400°F) oven (180°C/350°F fan-forced), turning occasionally and swapping the trays around on the oven shelves halfway through cooking, for 50–55 minutes or until the wings are cooked and deep golden. Serve sprinkled with 4 thinly sliced spring onions (scallions) and 2 tablespoons toasted sesame seeds.

Lamb stir-fry

Combine 700 g (1 lb 9 oz) lamb stir-fry strips with the marinade, then cover and chill for at least 2 hours or overnight to marinate. Heat a large non-stick wok over high heat. Stir-fry the lamb, in four batches, for 3 minutes each, until just cooked and golden. Serve on top of cooked noodles and steamed Asian greens.

Pork noodles

In a large non-stick wok over high heat, stir-fry 700 g (1 lb 9 oz) minced (ground) pork for about 10 minutes or until cooked and golden. Add the marinade, then stir-fry for 5 minutes or until thickened and sticky. Serve over shelf-ready soba noodles and top with thinly sliced spring onion (scallion) and julienned Lebanese (short) cucumber.

Moroccan marinade

makes approximately 350 g (12 oz/1¾ cups)
preparation 10 minutes

15 g (½ oz/½ cup) coriander (cilantro) leaves
10 g (¼ oz/½ cup) flat-leaf (Italian) parsley leaves
2 tablespoons Moroccan spice blend (page 25)
125 ml (4 fl oz/½ cup) red wine vinegar
185 ml (6 fl oz/¾ cup) avocado oil

1 Add the coriander and parsley to the mixer bowl, measuring cup in. Chop for 3 sec/speed 7. Scrape down the side of the bowl.

2 Add the remaining ingredients to the mixer bowl, measuring cup in. Combine for 5 sec/speed 5.

TRY THIS

Rub over lamb backstrap (loin fillet) before barbecuing

Sprinkle over firm tofu before pan-frying

Sprinkle over roasted red onion wedges before adding to pasta salad

Toss through drained and rinsed tinned chickpeas

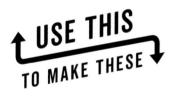

Barbecued corn

Combine 6 corn cobs and the marinade in a flat dish and leave to stand at room temperature for at least 2 hours, turning occasionally. Cook on a preheated barbecue chargrill plate on medium heat for 10–12 minutes, turning the cobs occasionally, until cooked and dark golden. Return the corn to the dish with the marinade and toss to recoat the corn in the mixture. Serve hot.

Slow-cooked beef

Combine the marinade, 700 g (1 lb 9 oz) chopped lean chuck steak, 3 quartered onions and 125 ml (4 fl oz/½ cup) water in a slow cooker on High. Cook, stirring occasionally, for 6 hours or until very tender and the sauce has reduced slightly. Serve with rice.

Moroccan couscous

Combine 475 g (1 lb 1 oz/2½ cups) couscous, the marinade and 125 ml (4 fl oz/½ cup) boiling water in a large heatproof bowl. Immediately cover tightly with plastic wrap and stand for around 10 minutes or until the couscous has absorbed all the liquid and is tender. Using a fork, fluff to separate the grains. Add 400 g (14 oz) drained and rinsed tinned chickpeas and 1 bunch thinly sliced radishes. Toss to combine. Serve with your pan-fried protein of choice.

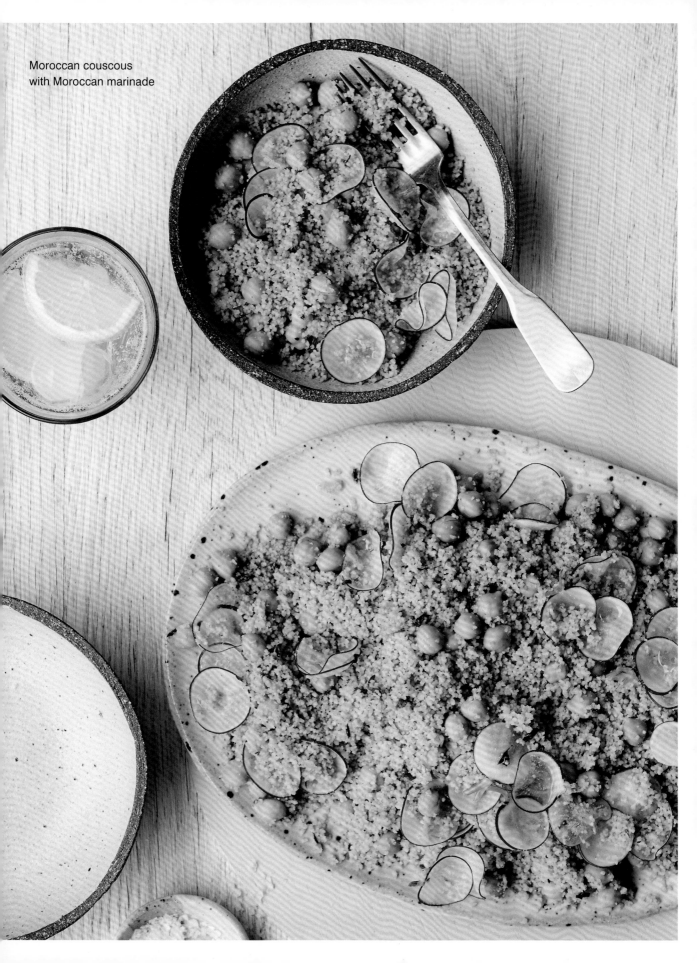

Moroccan couscous
with Moroccan marinade

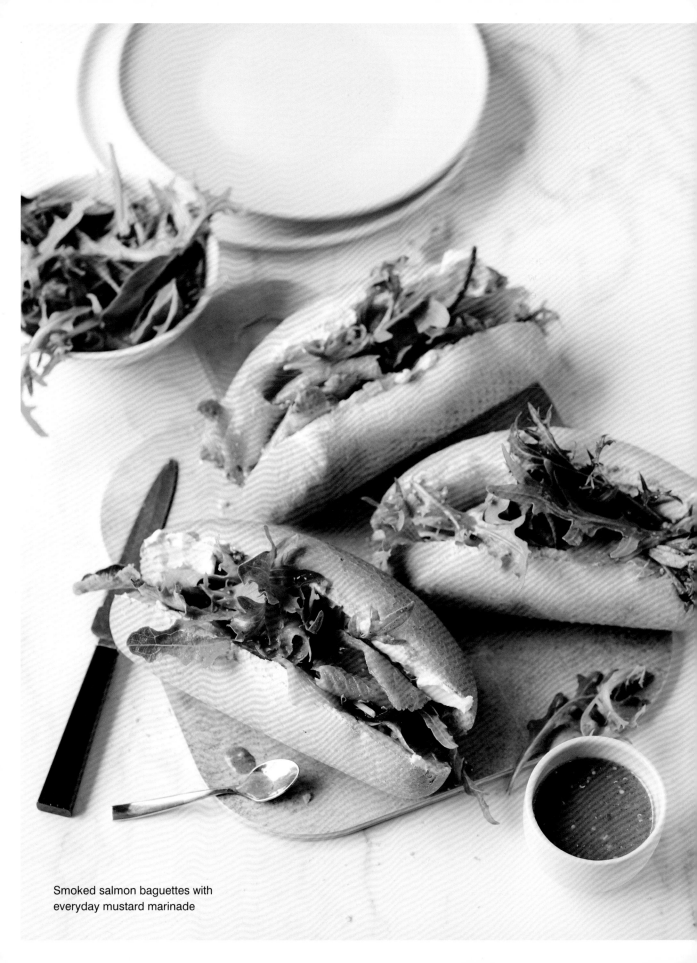

Smoked salmon baguettes with
everyday mustard marinade

Everyday mustard marinade

makes approximately 320 g (11¼ oz/1½ cups)
preparation 10 minutes

2 garlic cloves
1 tablespoon All-purpose spice blend (page 22)
2 tablespoons wholegrain mustard
125 ml (4 fl oz/½ cup) white wine vinegar
185 ml (6 fl oz/¾ cup) extra virgin olive oil
2 tablespoons chopped chives

1 Add the garlic to the mixer bowl, measuring cup in. Chop for 3 sec/speed 7. Scrape down the side of the bowl.

2 Add the remaining ingredients to the mixer bowl, measuring cup in. Combine for 5 sec/speed 5.

TRY THIS

Use as a post-cooking marinade for chargrilled steaks

Stir through drained and rinsed tinned lentils and steamed mixed vegies

Makes a great dressing for Caesar salad

Use to marinate cooked peeled prawns (shrimp) before making a prawn cocktail salad

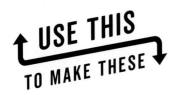
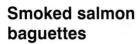

USE THIS TO MAKE THESE

Smoked salmon baguettes

Split 6 white baguette rolls in half and spread each with 1 tablespoon spreadable cream cheese. Fill the rolls evenly with mixed salad leaves, then 300 g (10½ oz) sliced smoked salmon. Drizzle with 105 g (3½ oz/½ cup) of the marinade, then serve.

Roast vegies

Combine 2 chopped onions, 4 chopped carrots, 4 chopped zucchini (courgettes), 1 chopped head of broccoli, 1 chopped small head of cauliflower and the marinade together in a large, deep roasting tin. Toss well to combine and coat. Roast in a preheated 200°C (400°F) oven (180°C/350°F fan-forced) for 45–50 minutes, tossing occasionally or until cooked and golden. Serve with your roasted or pan-fried protein of choice.

Pork cutlets with salad

Combine 2 shaved baby fennel bulbs; 200 g (7 oz) mixed salad leaves; 1 red apple, cut into very thin wedges; 1 red onion, cut into very thin wedges and 210 g (7½ oz/ 1 cup) of the marinade in a bowl. Chargrill 6 pork cutlets over medium–high heat for 12 minutes or until cooked and golden. Serve with the salad.

Italian balsamic marinade

makes approximately 420 g (15 oz/1⅔ cups)
preparation 10 minutes

3 garlic cloves
15 g (½ oz/½ cup) basil
  leaves
2 tablespoons Italian spice
  blend (page 14)

125 ml (4 fl oz/½ cup) extra
  virgin olive oil
185 ml (6 fl oz/¾ cup)
  balsamic vinegar
2 tablespoons honey

1 Add the garlic and basil to the mixer bowl, measuring cup in. Chop
   for 3 sec/speed 7. Scrape down the side of the bowl.

2 Add the remaining ingredients to the mixer bowl, measuring cup in.
   Combine for 5 sec/speed 5.

TRY THIS

Sprinkle over eggplant
(aubergine) halves before
barbecuing, pastry parcels of
feta cheese before chargrilling,
mixed chopped winter vegies
before roasting, or crisp rocket
(arugula) leaves

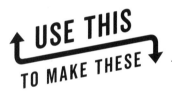

USE THIS TO MAKE THESE

Chicken skewers

Sprinkle the marinade over 700 g
(1 lb 9 oz) chicken tenderloins.
Thread the chicken onto 12 metal
skewers and chill for at least 1 hour
before chargrilling for 8–10 minutes
over medium heat. Serve with
salad or vegetables.

Salmon caprese

Pan-fry 6 x 120 g (4¼ oz) skinless,
boneless salmon portions in
a large non-stick frying pan for
3 minutes on each side for
medium, or cook to your liking.
Add the fish to a large heatproof
bowl and thickly flake with a fork.
Add 150 g (5½ oz) baby spinach
(English spinach) leaves; 1 small
bunch basil leaves, picked; 300 g
(10½ oz) torn baby bocconcini
(fresh baby mozzarella cheese);
1 thinly sliced red onion; 6 thinly
sliced vine-ripened tomatoes and
the marinade. Serve.

Tomato bruschetta

Toss the marinade through
700 g (1 lb 9 oz) chopped mixed
tomatoes and leave to stand for
at least 1 hour. Use to top
6 large chargrilled slices of pide
(Turkish/flat bread).

Indian yoghurt marinade

makes approximately 450 g (1 lb/1¾ cups)
preparation 10 minutes

10 g (¼ oz/½ cup) mint leaves
2 tablespoons Madras paste
  (page 127)
260 g (9¼ oz/1 cup) plain
  Greek-style yoghurt

60 ml (2 fl oz/¼ cup)
  red wine vinegar
80 ml (2½ fl oz/⅓ cup)
  avocado oil

1 Add the mint to the mixer bowl, measuring cup in. Chop for 3 sec/
   speed 7. Scrape down the side of the bowl.

2 Add the remaining ingredients to the mixer bowl, measuring cup in.
   Combine for 5 sec/speed 5.

TRY THIS

Drizzle over chargrilled steak
as a sauce

Use as a dip for roasted vegies

Rub over raw prawns (shrimp)
before barbecuing

**Sprinkle over zucchini
(courgettes) before roasting**

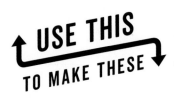

USE THIS TO MAKE THESE

Tofu toss

On medium–high heat, chargrill
700 g (1 lb 9 oz) sliced firm tofu
and 2 bunches trimmed broccolini
for 5–7 minutes, or until heated
through and dark golden. Transfer
to a large heatproof bowl and add
the marinade. Toss well to coat.
Serve over mixed salad greens
and sliced cucumber.

Grilled salmon

Combine 6 x 200 g (7 oz) skinless,
boneless salmon portions and the
marinade in a flat glass or ceramic
dish. Turn to coat well in the
mixture. Cover and chill for 2 hours
to marinate. Preheat a grill (broiler)
to high. Add the salmon to a
foil-lined and greased baking tray.
Cook under the grill for 12 minutes,
turning carefully just once, for
medium, or cook to your liking.
Serve with steamed vegies and
lime wedges.

Chicken wraps

Combine the marinade and 700 g
(1 lb 9 oz) small skinless chicken
thigh fillets in a bowl. Chill for at
least 2 hours or overnight. Preheat
a barbecue flatplate to medium.
Cook the chicken, turning the meat
occasionally, for 18–20 minutes or
until cooked and golden. Rest for
5 minutes before roughly pulling the
meat apart and serving it on top of
3 Lebanese (short) cucumbers, cut
into ribbons using a peeler; 1 bunch
baby carrots; 120 g (4¼ oz/2 cups)
shredded iceberg lettuce; 20 g
(¾ oz/1 cup) small mint leaves and
25 g (1 oz/¼ cup) toasted flaked
almonds on lightly chargrilled soft,
wholemeal (whole-wheat) wraps.
Fold up to serve.

Zesty-mex marinade

makes approximately 240 g (8¾ oz/1 cup)
preparation 10 minutes

15 g (½ oz/½ cup) coriander (cilantro) leaves
2 tablespoons Mexican spice blend (page 18)
zest and juice of 4 large limes
125 ml (4 fl oz/½ cup) avocado oil

1 Add the coriander to the mixer bowl, measuring cup in. Chop for
3 sec/speed 7. Scrape down the side of the bowl.

2 Add the remaining ingredients to the mixer bowl, measuring cup in.
Combine for 5 sec/speed 5.

TRY THIS

Use as a dressing for an
avocado and iceberg salad

**Add to red onion wedges
before barbecuing**

Use to season a sweet potato
and black bean smash

**Use to marinate pork ribs
before roasting**

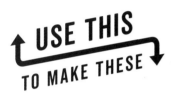

Pulled pork

Cut 700 g (1 lb 9 oz) lean pork
shoulder into 3 cm (1¼ inch) pieces
and add to a slow cooker with the
marinade and 400 g (14 oz) tinned
chopped tomatoes. Cook on High
for 6 hours or until the pork is
falling apart and the sauce has
reduced. Using two forks, shred
the pork meat. Serve in toasted
brioche rolls along with a store-
bought shredded coleslaw mix
and sliced jalapeños. Dress with
lime juice and serve.

Beef tacos

Brown 700 g (1 lb 9 oz) minced
(ground) beef in a large, deep
non-stick frying pan over high
heat for 10 minutes until cooked
and deep golden. Remove the pan
from the heat. Add the marinade
and stir to combine. Spoon the
mixture into baked taco shells, then
top with crumbled Danish feta
cheese, finely shredded iceberg
lettuce and thinly sliced spring
onions (scallions). Serve.

Eggplant steaks

Cut 3 eggplants (aubergines)
in half lengthways and score
the skin. Cook on a preheated
barbecue chargrill plate on
high for 15–18 minutes, turning
occasionally, until softened and
caramelised. Transfer to a flat
ceramic glass dish, cut side up.
Pour over the marinade and stand
for 10 minutes. Serve topped with
diced avocado and coriander
(cilantro) leaves.

Classic French marinade

makes approximately 350 g (12 oz/1¾ cups)
preparation 10 minutes

2 tablespoons French spice blend (page 21)
1 tablespoon dijon mustard
juice of 2 lemons
185 ml (6 fl oz/¾ cup) extra virgin olive oil
20 g (¾ oz/⅓ cup) chervil leaves

Add all the ingredients to the mixer bowl, measuring cup in. Combine for 5 sec/speed 5.

TRY THIS

Use to dress a crisp green salad

Toss through roasted kipfler (fingerling) potatoes

Use to marinate asparagus before lightly steaming

Rub over snapper fillets before pan-frying

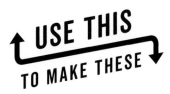

USE THIS TO MAKE THESE

French potato bake

Place 1 kg (2 lb 4 oz) all-purpose potatoes, peeled and very thinly sliced, in a bowl. Add the marinade, 250 ml (9 fl oz/1 cup) thin (pouring/whipping) cream and 150 g (5½ oz) crumbled aged cheddar cheese. Toss to ensure all the potato is covered in the mixture. Layer the mixture in a large, heavy-based, buttered baking dish. Cover with a piece of baking paper, then doubled pieces of foil, tightly wrapped. Bake in a preheated 200°C (400°F) oven (180°C/350°F fan-forced) for 1 hour 20 minutes or until the potatoes are tender. Bake, uncovered, for 20 minutes more or until the top is golden and crisp. Stand for 5 minutes before serving with your roasted, grilled or barbecued protein of choice.

Chicken and asparagus

Place the marinade in a large, flat ceramic or glass dish. Cook 700 g (1 lb 9 oz) chicken tenderloins and 2 bunches trimmed asparagus under a grill (broiler) on high for 10 minutes, turning occasionally, or until cooked and light golden. Immediately transfer the chicken and asparagus to the dish with the marinade, turning to coat well. Stand for 5 minutes to marinate, then add 50 g (1¾ oz) baby rocket (arugula) leaves. Toss well to combine, then serve.

Salmon niçoise

Cook 6 eggs in a saucepan of boiling water for 3 minutes for soft-boiled, or cook to your liking. Immediately transfer the eggs to a bowl of iced water to chill. Peel, then halve the eggs lengthways. In a larger bowl, combine the marinade; 830 g (1 lb 13 oz) tinned red salmon, drained and flaked; 500 g (1 lb 2 oz) baby green beans, blanched and trimmed; 700 g (1 lb 9 oz) cooked baby potatoes, halved; 3 baby cos (romaine) lettuces, leaves separated; 200 g (7 oz) medley baby tomatoes, halved and 100 g (3½ oz) pitted kalamata olives. Gently toss to combine and coat well. Divide among serving plates. Serve topped with the egg halves.

8-week menu plan

Welcome to your 8-week menu plan, where all you need to do is set aside some time on a Sunday to prep for all your Monday–Wednesday night dinners. Yep, that's three nights sorted. I make this easy for you with Sunday prep guides and shopping lists for each week. After your 'super' Sunday, you'll have one meal cooked in full so all you have to do is reheat it, and two meals prepped to the point where you just need to finish them off, so you can get your meals on the table quickly and with minimal fuss. The meals make great use of the simple spice blends and marinades at the beginning of this chapter and, of course, your thermo appliance will be working hard for you.

These pre-prepped meals will be like gold for those days when the house is in chaos mode, in the midst of schoolday/workday routines and afternoon parent-taxi runs. And because I've given you eight weeks of options, you'll have plenty of variety. Follow along each week, or select a week or two and put them on repeat.

Each of the recipes in this chapter serves 6 to suit larger families, those with super-hungry teens, or to allow for leftovers you can chill overnight for lunch the next day. All recipes use eight ingredients or less, recipe cooking or re-heating times are kept to 30 minutes or under, and I utilise some great supermarket grab-and-go's too.

HERE'S YOUR 8-WEEK MENU PLAN AT A GLANCE

Each week's meal plan has a Sunday prep guide for you to follow, so all you have to do is check your pantry and fridge to see what you may already have prepped, then whip up the rest. I've also organised a shopping list for the start of each week, so simply grab your phone, take a quick photo of the list, then head to the shops!

	Week 1	Week 2	Week 3	Week 4
Mon	Moroccan chicken and couscous	Sweet soy beef steaks	Zesty-mex pork and vegie rice	Beef sausages and Thai potato salad
Tues	French-roasted salmon and potatoes	Chicken korma tenderloins	Tuna lasagne	Italian balsamic chicken tray bake
Wed	Vegie dal	Thai prawn stir-fry	Chinese beef and vegie stir-fry	Moroccan tofu and couscous salad

	Week 5	Week 6	Week 7	Week 8
Mon	Beef and overnight noodles	Flathead bistro salad with orange	Everyday beef and vegie skewers	Pork naan
Tues	Indian chickpea stuffed sweet potatoes	Bean minestrone	Creamy tuna ravioli	Moroccan beef meatball and chickpea bake
Wed	Chicken sausage and coleslaw tortillas	Chinese tofu and egg noodles	Warm Thai chicken and rice noodle salad	Antipasto pasta

week 1

Shopping list

Fruit & veg

- [ ] 2 red capsicums (peppers)
- [ ] 3 lemons
- [ ] 2 limes
- [ ] 3 zucchini (courgettes)
- [ ] 100 g (3½ oz) baby spinach (English spinach) leaves
- [ ] 1 kg (2 lb 4 oz) baby potatoes
- [ ] 2 large leeks
- [ ] 2 bunches asparagus
- [ ] 2 bunches chives
- [ ] 1 bunch coriander (cilantro)
- [ ] 1 bunch mint
- [ ] 1 onion

Protein

- [ ] 700 g (1 lb 9 oz) chicken stir-fry strips
- [ ] 6 x 180 g (6½ oz) skinless, boneless salmon portions

Pantry items

- [ ] 240 g (8¾ oz/1¼ cups) couscous
- [ ] 85 g (3 oz/½ cup) sultanas (golden raisins)
- [ ] 375 ml (13 fl oz/1½ cups) chicken stock
- [ ] 60 ml (2 fl oz/¼ cup) extra virgin olive oil
- [ ] 205 g (7¼ oz/1 cup) dried split red lentils
- [ ] 500 ml (17 fl oz/2 cups) vegetable stock
- [ ] naan

Fridge & freezer items

- [ ] 250 g (9 oz) butter
- [ ] 215 g (7½ oz/1½ cups) frozen pea, corn and red capsicum (pepper) mix
- [ ] raita

Plus your prepped Flavour Staples

- [ ] 1 full quantity Moroccan marinade (page 30)
- [ ] 1 tablespoon French spice blend (page 21)
- [ ] 2 tablespoons Indian spice blend (page 17)

Sunday prep guide

MEAL 1

FOR MONDAY

MOROCCAN CHICKEN AND COUSCOUS
(PAGE 42)

➡ **Prepare the recipe up to the end of Step 3, and store as directed.**

➡ When you are ready to serve this for dinner, simply continue with the recipe from Step 4.

MEAL 2

FOR TUESDAY

FRENCH-ROASTED SALMON AND POTATOES
(PAGE 45)

➡ **Prepare the recipe up to the end of Step 4, and store as directed.**

➡ When you are ready to serve this for dinner, simply reheat the dish as directed in Step 5.

MEAL 3

FOR WEDNESDAY

VEGIE DAL
(PAGE 46)

 Prepare the vegetables, then store them in an airtight container in the fridge.

 When you are ready to serve this for dinner, cook the recipe from Step 1.

Moroccan chicken and couscous

serves 6
preparation 25 minutes, plus 10 minutes standing time,
   plus overnight chilling time
cooking 12 minutes

1 full quantity Moroccan marinade (page 30)
700 g (1 lb 9 oz) chicken stir-fry strips
2 red capsicums (peppers), sliced
240 g (8¾ oz/1¼ cups) couscous
85 g (3 oz/½ cup) sultanas (golden raisins)
375 ml (13 fl oz/1½ cups) chicken stock
100 g (3½ oz) baby spinach (English spinach) leaves
mint sprigs, to serve
lemon cheeks, to serve

1 Place the marinade, chicken and capsicum in a large airtight container.
Stir well to combine and coat everything evenly in the marinade mixture.
Cover and chill overnight.

2 Place the couscous in a large heatproof bowl.

3 Add the sultanas and stock to the mixer bowl, measuring cup in.
Heat for 3 min/120°C/reverse stir/speed 1. Transfer the mixture to the
bowl with the couscous, stir with a fork, then immediately cover. Stand
for 10 minutes or until the couscous has absorbed the stock. Use a fork
to fluff and separate the grains. Cover and chill overnight.

4 Preheat a barbecue chargrill plate to medium–high. Remove the
couscous bowl from the fridge.

5 Cook the chicken and capsicum on the barbecue chargrill plate for
5–8 minutes, turning occasionally, or until cooked and golden. Transfer
to the bowl with the couscous, then add the spinach. Toss everything
together to combine and top with the mint. Serve with the lemon cheeks.

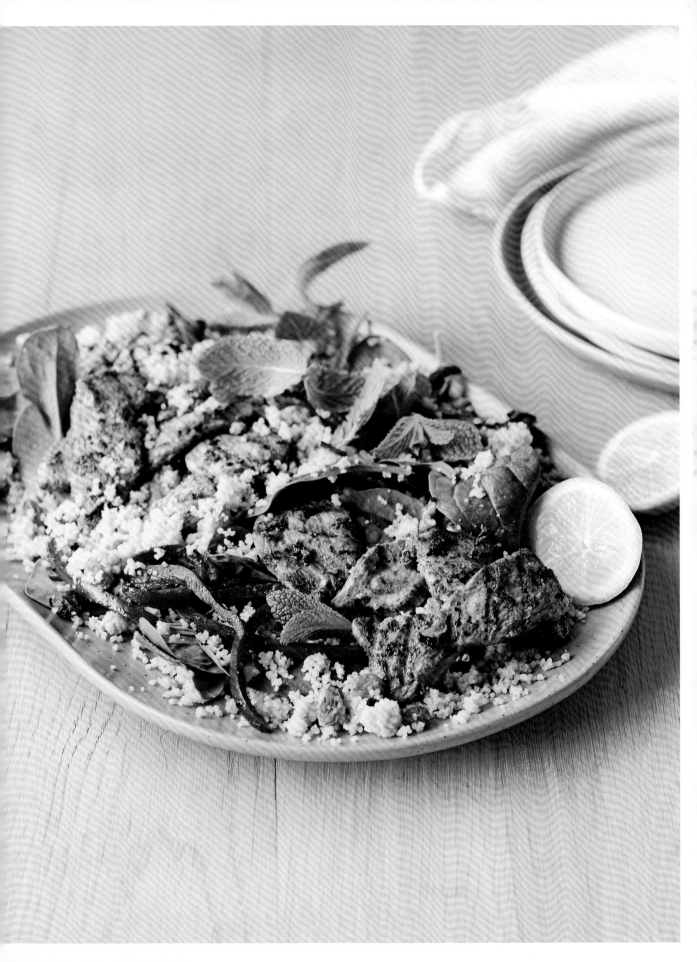

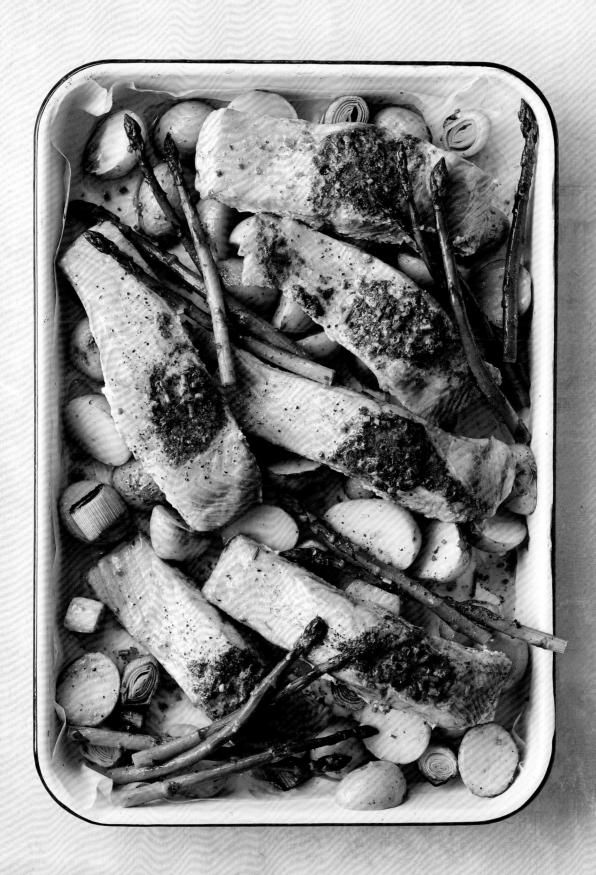

French-roasted salmon and potatoes

serves 6
preparation 30 minutes, plus cooling time,
 plus chilling time
cooking 40 minutes

60 ml (2 fl oz/¼ cup) extra virgin olive oil
1 kg (2 lb 4 oz) baby potatoes, halved
2 large leeks, white part only, thickly sliced
6 x 180 g (6½ oz) skinless, boneless salmon portions
2 bunches asparagus, trimmed
chopped chives, to serve (optional)

FRENCH-SPICED BUTTER
1 small bunch chives, finely chopped
1 tablespoon French spice blend (page 21)
juice of 2 lemons, with the rind cut into strips
250 g (9 oz) butter, at room temperature

1 Preheat the oven to 200°C (400°F)/180°C (350°F) fan-forced.

2 Add the oil, potatoes and leek to a large, heavy-based baking dish and toss well to coat. Roast in the oven, turning once, for 25 minutes or until just tender and crisp. Cool completely in the dish.

3 Meanwhile, make the French-spiced butter by adding all the ingredients to the mixer bowl, measuring cup in. Mix for 5 sec/speed 4. Scrape down the side of the bowl. Set aside.

4 Rest the salmon portions over the top of the cooled potato mixture in the dish, scatter with the asparagus then dollop over the French-spiced butter. Cover tightly with plastic wrap. Keep stored in the fridge for up to 2 days.

5 To serve, bring the dish out of the fridge and leave on the bench top while the oven preheats. Preheat the oven to 220°C (425°F)/200°C (400°F) fan-forced. Remove the plastic wrap from the dish, then roast for 15 minutes or until the vegetables are heated through and the salmon is cooked medium, or cook further to your liking. Serve straight to the table, sprinkled with the chopped chives, if using.

Vegie dal

serves 6
preparation 20 minutes
cooking 25 minutes

1 onion, quartered
3 zucchini (courgettes), cut into 2 cm (¾ inch) pieces
2 tablespoons Indian spice blend (page 17)
205 g (7¼ oz/1 cup) dried split red lentils
500 ml (17 fl oz/2 cups) vegetable stock
215 g (7½ oz/1½ cups) frozen pea, corn and
  red capsicum (pepper) mix
coriander (cilantro) leaves, to serve
6 naan, toasted, to serve
lime wedges, to serve
raita, to serve

1 Add the onion and zucchini to the mixer bowl, measuring cup in.
  Chop for 5 sec/speed 7. Scrape down the side of the bowl. Chop for
  5 sec/speed 7. Scrape down the side of the bowl. Cook for 10 min/
  100°C/speed 1. Scrape down the side of the bowl.

2 Add the spice blend, lentils and stock to the mixer bowl, measuring
  cup in. Cook for 12 min/100°C/reverse stir/speed 1.

3 Add the frozen vegetables to the mixer bowl, measuring cup in.
  Cook for 3 min/80°C/reverse stir/speed 1. Serve the dal sprinkled
  with the coriander, with the naan, lime wedges and raita alongside.

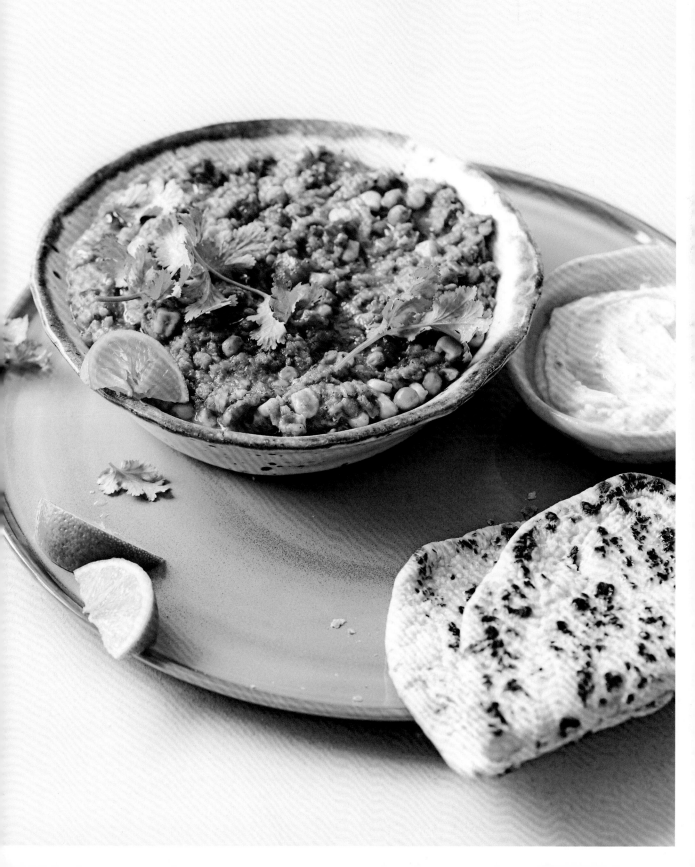

week 2

Shopping list

Fruit & veg

- [ ] 2 limes
- [ ] 5 cm (2 inch) piece fresh ginger
- [ ] 2 garlic cloves
- [ ] 7 spring onions (scallions)
- [ ] 800 g (1 lb 12 oz) store-bought fresh stir-fry vegetable mix (broccoli, red cabbage, onion, snow pea/mangetout, carrot, zucchini/courgette, capsicum/pepper)
- [ ] 1 red onion
- [ ] 500 g (1 lb 2 oz) orange sweet potatoes
- [ ] 500 g (1 lb 2 oz) sugar snap peas
- [ ] 1 bunch Thai basil

- [ ] 1 bunch coriander (cilantro)
- [ ] 100 g (3½ oz) baby spinach (English spinach) leaves

Protein

- [ ] 6 x 150 g (5½ oz) beef fillet steaks
- [ ] 700 g (1 lb 9 oz) chicken tenderloins
- [ ] 700 g (1 lb 9 oz) peeled, deveined raw prawns (shrimp)

Pantry items

- [ ] 2 tablespoons macadamia oil
- [ ] 400 g (14 oz) tinned chopped tomatoes

- [ ] shelf-ready basmati rice
- [ ] 2 teaspoons brown sugar
- [ ] 225 g (8 oz) tinned sliced bamboo shoots
- [ ] dried rice vermicelli noodles

Fridge & freezer items

- [ ] hokkien (egg) noodles

Plus your prepped Flavour Staples

- [ ] 1 full quantity Sweet soy marinade (page 29)
- [ ] 1 full quantity Korma paste (page 127)
- [ ] 1 full quantity Thai spiced marinade (page 26)

Sunday prep guide

MEAL 1

FOR MONDAY

SWEET SOY BEEF STEAKS
(PAGE 50)

 Prepare the recipe up to the end of Step 2, and store as directed.

→ When you are ready to serve this for dinner, simply continue with the recipe from Step 3.

MEAL 2

FOR TUESDAY

CHICKEN KORMA TENDERLOINS
(PAGE 53)

 Prepare the recipe up to the end of Step 4, and store as directed.

→ When you are ready to serve this for dinner, simply reheat the dish as directed in Step 5.

MEAL 3

FOR WEDNESDAY

THAI PRAWN STIR-FRY
(PAGE 54)

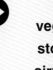 **Prepare the vegetables, then store them in an airtight container in the fridge.**

 When you are ready to serve this for dinner, cook the recipe from Step 1.

Sweet soy beef steaks

serves 6
preparation 40 minutes, plus overnight chilling time
cooking 10 minutes

1 full quantity Sweet soy marinade (page 29)
6 x 150 g (5½ oz) beef fillet steaks
5 cm (2 inch) piece fresh ginger, peeled
  and halved
2 garlic cloves
4 spring onions (scallions), cut into 2 cm
  (¾ inch) pieces, plus 1 extra thinly sliced
2 tablespoons macadamia oil
800 g (1 lb 12 oz) store-bought fresh mixed
  traditional stir-fry vegetables (such as broccoli,
  red cabbage, onion, snow peas/mangetout,
  carrot, zucchini/courgette, red capsicum/pepper)
hokkien (egg) noodles, to serve

1 Place the marinade and beef in a bowl. Stir well to combine and
  coat the meat evenly in the marinade mixture. Transfer to an airtight
  container and cover with any remaining marinade from the bowl.
  Cover and chill overnight.

2 Add the ginger, garlic, spring onion and oil to the mixer bowl, measuring
  cup in. Chop for 5 sec/speed 7. Scrape down the side of the bowl.
  Chop for 5 sec/speed 7. Scrape down the side of the bowl. Transfer the
  mixture to an airtight container. Add the stir-fry vegetables. Toss to
  combine and coat evenly in the oil mixture. Cover and chill overnight.

3 Preheat a barbecue chargrill plate and barbecue flatplate to high.

4 Cook the beef on the barbecue chargrill plate, and the vegetable
  mixture on the barbecue flatplate for 5–8 minutes, turning occasionally,
  or until cooked and golden. Serve with the noodles, topped with the
  extra thinly sliced spring onion.

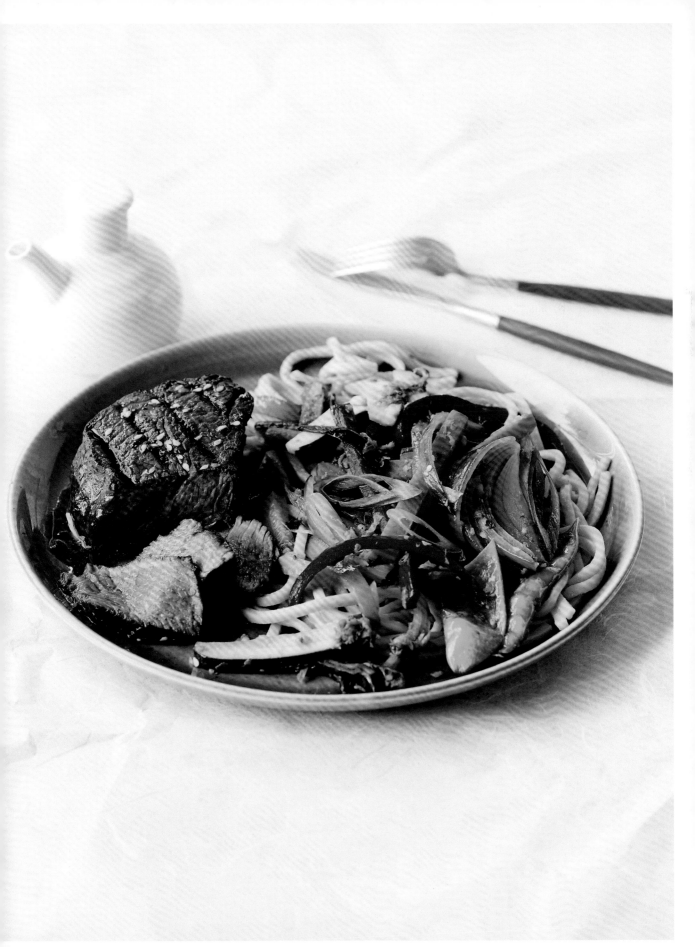

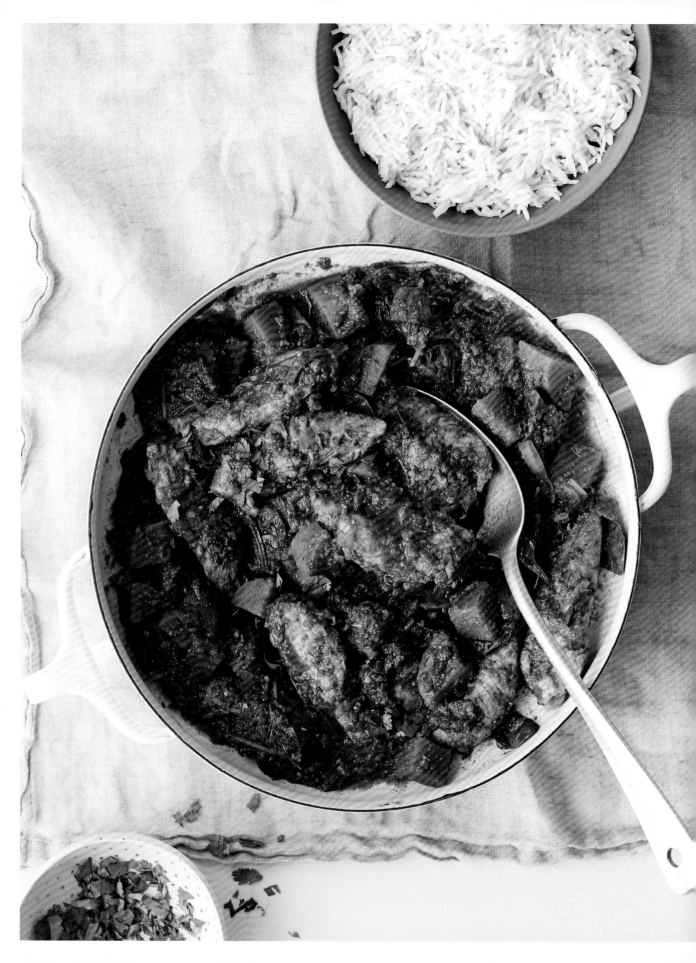

Chicken korma tenderloins

serves 6
preparation 20 minutes, plus cooling time,
  plus chilling time, plus 10 minutes standing time
cooking 40 minutes

1 red onion, quartered
400 g (14 oz) tinned chopped tomatoes
½ quantity Korma paste (page 127)
700 g (1 lb 9 oz) chicken tenderloins
500 g (1 lb 2 oz) orange sweet potatoes,
  peeled and chopped
100 g (3½ oz) baby spinach (English spinach) leaves
chopped coriander (cilantro), to serve
cooked basmati rice, to serve

1 Add the onion to the mixer bowl, measuring cup in. Chop for
   10 sec/speed 7. Scrape down the side of the bowl.

2 Add the tomatoes to the mixer bowl, measuring cup in. Cook
   for 5 min/100°C/speed 1.

3 Transfer the mixture to a large, deep, heavy-based frying pan over
   medium heat. Add the paste, chicken and sweet potato to the pan.
   Stir until the mixture comes to a simmer. Reduce the heat to low.
   Cover and simmer gently, stirring occasionally, for 15 minutes or
   until cooked and the sauce is reduced slightly. Remove from the
   heat, cool the mixture in the pan. Add the spinach and stir to combine,
   then cover with a lid.

4 Transfer the pan to the fridge and chill for up to 2 days.

5 To serve, remove the pan from the fridge and leave to stand for
   10 minutes. Reheat the mixture in the pan over medium–low heat
   for 15 minutes, stirring occasionally and adding a little water if needed
   to loosen, or until heated. Serve sprinkled with the coriander, and the
   rice alongside.

Thai prawn stir-fry

serves 6
preparation 20 minutes
cooking 20 minutes

2 spring onions (scallions), cut into 2 cm
  (¾ inch) pieces
2 teaspoons brown sugar
1 full quantity Thai spiced marinade (page 26)
700 g (1 lb 9 oz) peeled, deveined raw
  prawns (shrimp), tails left on
500 g (1 lb 2 oz) sugar snap peas, trimmed
225 g (8 oz) tinned sliced bamboo shoots, drained and rinsed
soaked dried rice vermicelli noodles, to serve
Thai basil leaves, to serve
lime cheeks, to serve

1 Add the spring onion and sugar to the mixer bowl, measuring cup in.
   Chop for 5 sec/speed 7. Scrape down the side of the bowl.

2 Transfer the mixture to a bowl. Add the marinade and prawns. Toss
   to combine and coat well in the mixture.

3 Heat a large non-stick wok over high heat. Stir-fry the prawns, in four
   batches, for 3–4 minutes each or until just cooked and light golden.
   Transfer to a bowl.

4 Add the sugar snap peas and bamboo shoots to the same wok,
   along with 2 tablespoons water. Stir-fry for 2 minutes or until just
   tender. Return all the prawns to the wok. Toss together to combine.
   Serve immediately with the noodles, sprinkled with the Thai basil,
   and the lime cheeks alongside.

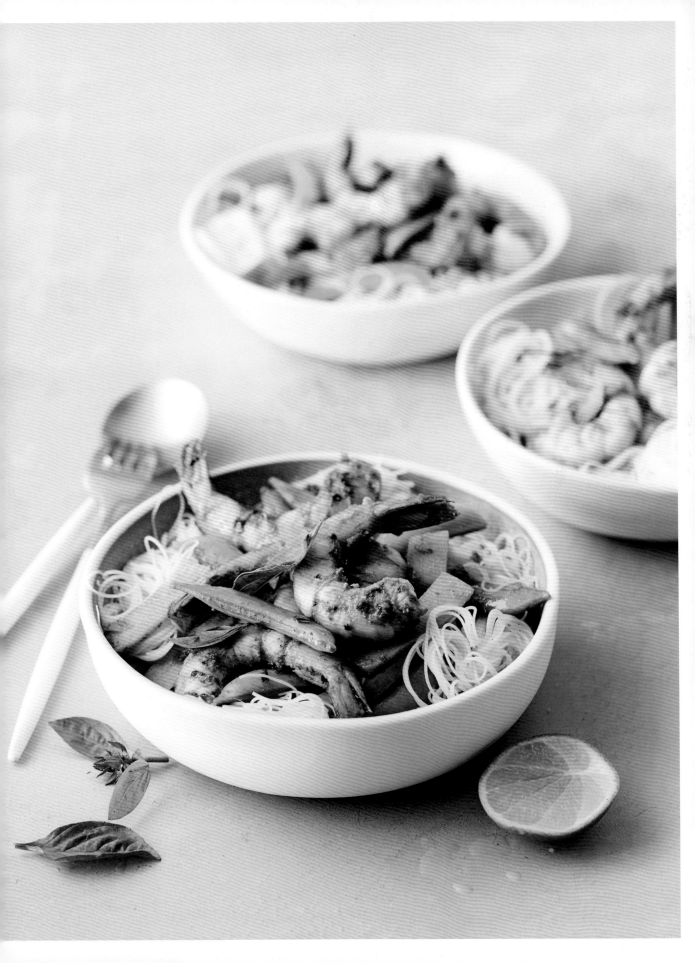

week 3

Shopping list

Fruit & veg

- [ ] 2 green capsicums (peppers)
- [ ] 2 zucchini (courgettes)
- [ ] 100 g (3½ oz) baby spinach (English spinach) leaves
- [ ] 4 carrots
- [ ] mixed salad leaves
- [ ] 250 g (9 oz) baby corn
- [ ] 1 bunch coriander (cilantro)
- [ ] 1 bunch flat-leaf (Italian) parsley
- [ ] 2 spring onions (scallions)

Protein

- [ ] 6 pork leg steaks
- [ ] 700 g (1 lb 9 oz) beef stir-fry strips

Pantry items

- [ ] 60 ml (2 fl oz/¼ cup) avocado oil
- [ ] 3 teaspoons smoked paprika
- [ ] 900 g (2 lb) shelf-ready long-grain white rice
- [ ] 850 g (1 lb 14 oz) tinned tuna in olive oil
- [ ] 800 g (1 lb 12 oz) store-bought red wine and garlic pasta sauce
- [ ] 375 g (13 oz) large instant dried lasagne sheets
- [ ] 2 tablespoons honey

Fridge & freezer items

- [ ] 285 g (10¼ oz/2 cups) frozen pea, corn and carrot mix
- [ ] sour cream
- [ ] 250 ml (9 fl oz/1 cup) cream for cooking
- [ ] 180 g (6½ oz/1½ cups) grated three-cheese mix (mozzarella, cheddar and parmesan)
- [ ] thin hokkien (egg) noodles

Plus your prepped Flavour Staples

- [ ] 1 full quantity Zesty-mex marinade (page 36)
- [ ] 2 tablespoons Chinese spice blend (page 24)

Sunday prep guide

FOR MONDAY

ZESTY-MEX PORK AND VEGIE RICE
(PAGE 58)

→ **Prepare the recipe up to the end of Step 1, and store as directed.**

→ When you are ready to serve this for dinner, just preheat a frying pan, then continue with the recipe from Step 2.

FOR TUESDAY

TUNA LASAGNE
(PAGE 61)

→ **Prepare the recipe up to the end of Step 5, and store as directed.**

→ When you are ready to serve this for dinner, simply reheat the dish as directed in Step 6.

FOR WEDNESDAY

CHINESE BEEF AND VEGIE STIR-FRY
(PAGE 62)

→ **Prepare the vegetables, then store them in an airtight container in the fridge.**

→ When you are ready to serve this for dinner, cook the recipe from Step 1.

Zesty-mex pork and vegie rice

serves 6
preparation 15 minutes, plus overnight chilling time
cooking 20 minutes

1 full quantity Zesty-mex marinade (page 36)
6 pork leg steaks
60 ml (2 fl oz/¼ cup) avocado oil
3 teaspoons smoked paprika
285 g (10¼ oz/2 cups) frozen pea, corn and carrot mix
900 g (2 lb) shelf-ready long-grain white rice
100 g (3½ oz) baby spinach (English spinach) leaves
coriander (cilantro) leaves, to serve
sour cream, to serve

1 Place the marinade and pork in a large airtight container. Stir well to combine and coat the meat evenly in the marinade mixture. Cover and chill overnight.

2 Heat a large, deep, non-stick frying pan over high heat. Cook the pork, turning only once, for 8–10 minutes or until cooked and golden. Transfer to a plate, cover loosely in foil and set aside.

3 Reheat the same pan over medium heat. Add the oil, paprika, vegetable mix and rice. Cook, tossing, for 5–8 minutes or until cooked and light golden. Remove the pan from the heat. Add the spinach. Toss together until well combined and the spinach just wilts.

4 Serve the rice mixture topped with the sliced pork and any resting juices, sprinkled with coriander, and a dollop of sour cream on the side.

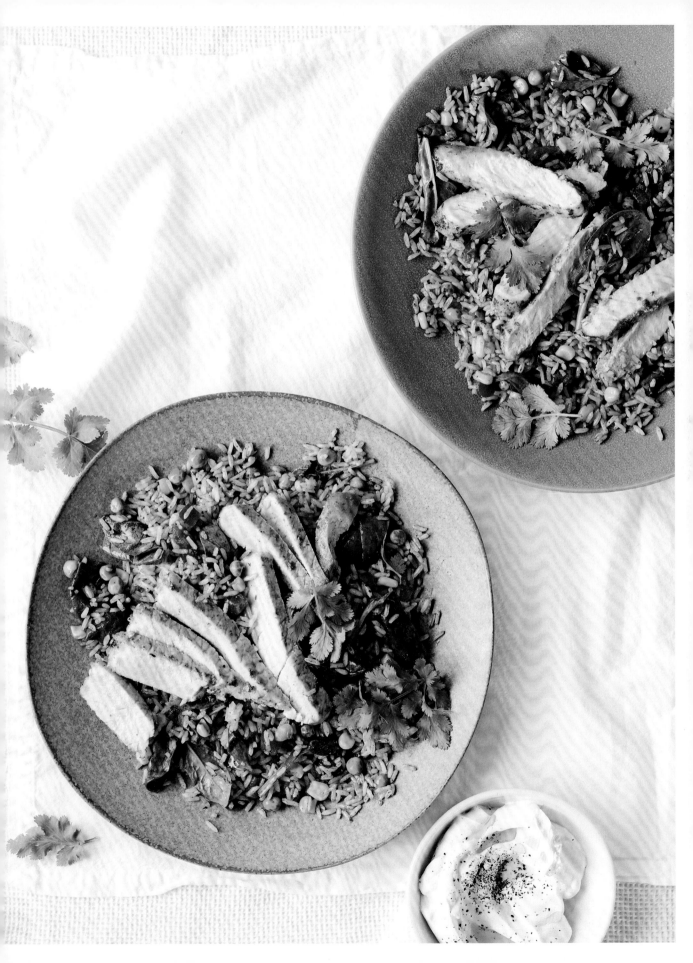

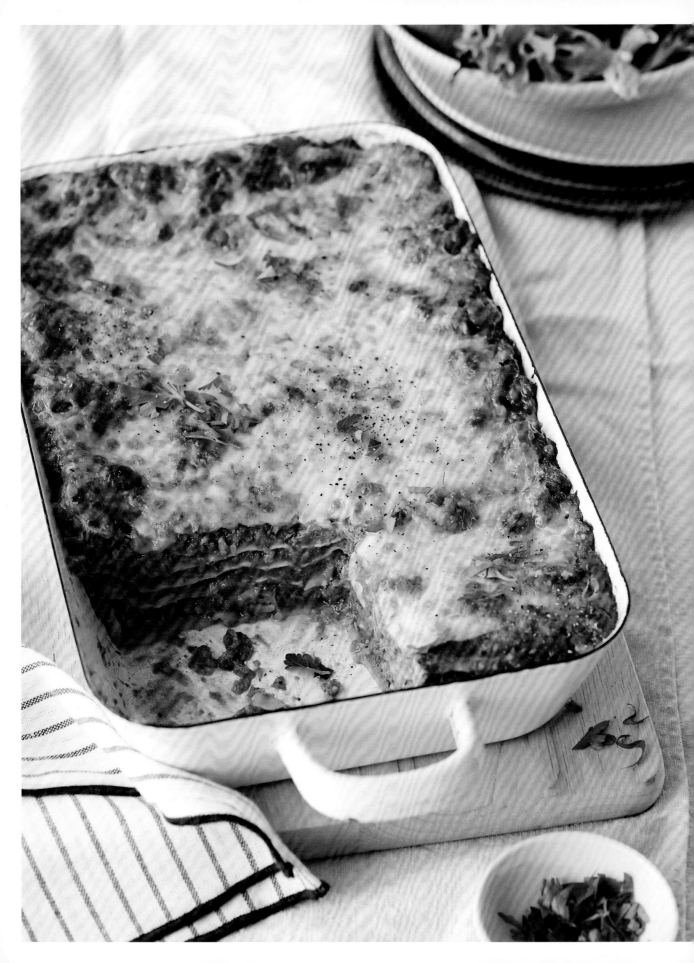

Tuna lasagne

serves 6
preparation 30 minutes, plus cooling time,
  plus chilling time
cooking 55 minutes

2 zucchini (courgettes), cut into 2 cm
  (¾ inch) pieces
2 carrots, cut into 2 cm (¾ inch) pieces
850 g (1 lb 14 oz) tinned tuna in olive oil
250 ml (9 fl oz/1 cup) cream for cooking
800 g (1 lb 12 oz) store-bought red wine
  and garlic pasta sauce
375 g (13 oz) instant dried large lasagne sheets
180 g (6½ oz/1½ cups) grated three-cheese mix
  (cheddar, parmesan and mozzarella)
chopped flat-leaf (Italian) parsley, to serve
mixed salad leaves, to serve

1 Preheat the oven to 200°C (400°F)/180°C (350°F) fan-forced.

2 Add the zucchini and carrot to the mixer bowl, measuring cup in.
   Chop for 5 sec/speed 7. Scrape down the side of the bowl. Chop
   for 5 sec/speed 7. Scrape down the side of the bowl.

3 Add the tuna and its oil, the cream and pasta sauce to the mixer
   bowl, measuring cup in. Mix for 10 sec/speed 4.

4 Layer the tuna mixture and lasagne sheets in a 30 x 20 x 7 cm
   (12 x 8 x 2¾ inch) baking dish, making sure to finish with a layer
   of the tuna mixture. Sprinkle with the cheese mix. Cover with a
   piece of baking paper, then cover tightly with a piece of foil. Bake
   in the oven for 30 minutes.

5 Remove from the oven. Cool completely while still covered with
   the foil. Remove the foil and discard. Cover tightly with plastic wrap,
   then store in the fridge for up to 2 days.

6 To serve, remove the dish from the fridge while the oven preheats.
   Preheat the oven to 200°C (400°F)/180°C (350°F) fan-forced.
   Remove the plastic wrap, then cover the dish tightly with foil. Bake
   for 15 minutes, remove the foil, then bake for 10 minutes more or
   until heated through and the top is golden and crisp. Serve sprinkled
   with the parsley, with the mixed salad alongside.

Chinese beef and vegie stir-fry

serves 6
preparation 20 minutes
cooking 15 minutes

2 tablespoons Chinese spice blend (page 24)
700 g (1 lb 9 oz) beef stir-fry strips
2 green capsicums (peppers), sliced
2 carrots, halved lengthways,
 then very thinly sliced diagonally
250 g (9 oz) baby corn, halved lengthways
2 tablespoons honey
sliced spring onion (scallion), to serve
thin hokkien (egg) noodles, to serve

1 Place the spice blend and beef in a bowl and toss well to combine and coat evenly.

2 Heat a large non-stick wok over high heat.

3 Stir-fry the beef mixture, in four batches, for 2–3 minutes each or until just cooked and golden. Transfer to a bowl.

4 Add the vegetables and honey to the wok with 60 ml (2 fl oz/¼ cup) water, then stir-fry for 2 minutes or until just tender and the water has reduced by half. Return all the beef to the wok and toss to combine. Serve sprinkled with the spring onion, with the noodles alongside.

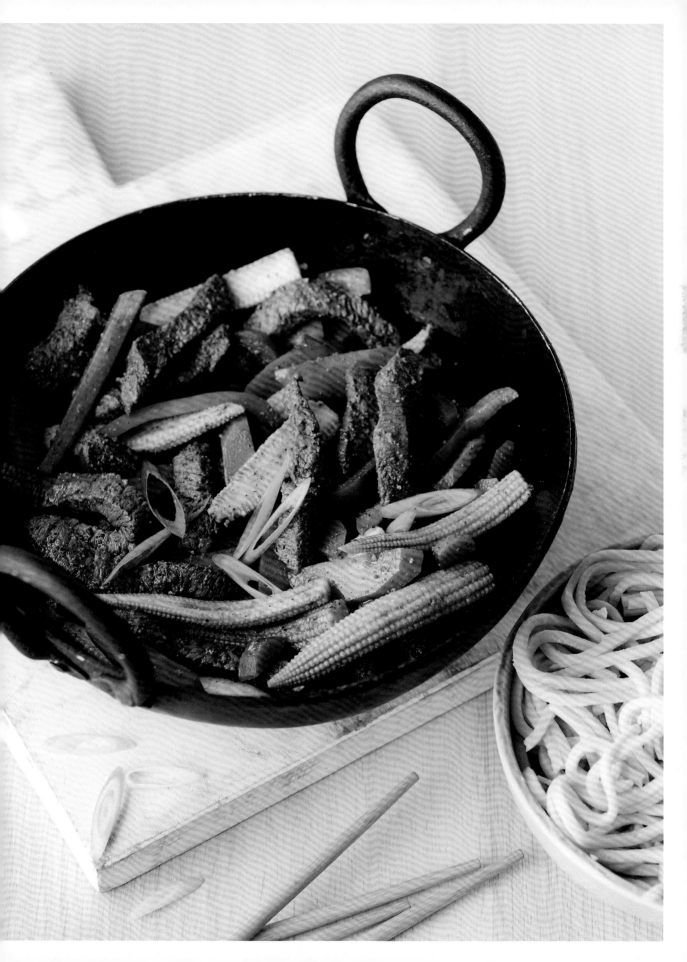

week 4

Shopping list

Fruit & veg

- [ ] 1 lemon
- [ ] 1 kg (2 lb 4 oz) cherry tomatoes
- [ ] 3 zucchini (courgettes)
- [ ] 3 Lebanese (short) cucumbers
- [ ] 4 celery stalks
- [ ] 2 carrots
- [ ] 4 spring onions (scallions)
- [ ] 1 kg (2 lb 4 oz) washed potatoes
- [ ] 1 bunch coriander (cilantro)
- [ ] 2 red onions
- [ ] 200 g (7 oz) baby rocket (arugula) leaves

Protein

- [ ] 12 thin beef sausages
- [ ] 700 g (1 lb 9 oz) diced skinless chicken breast fillets
- [ ] 700 g (1 lb 9 oz) firm tofu
- [ ] 4 eggs

Pantry items

- [ ] ciabatta loaf
- [ ] 240 g (8¾ oz/1¼ cups) couscous
- [ ] 375 ml (13 fl oz/1½ cups) vegetable stock

Fridge & freezer items

- [ ] 300 g (10½ oz) light sour cream
- [ ] parmesan cheese shavings

Plus your prepped Flavour Staples

- [ ] 2 tablespoons Thai spice blend (page 23)
- [ ] 1 full quantity Italian balsamic marinade (page 34)
- [ ] 1 full quantity Moroccan marinade (page 30)

SUN
DAY

Sunday prep guide

MEAL 1
FOR MONDAY

BEEF SAUSAGES AND THAI POTATO SALAD
(PAGE 66)

➡ **Prepare the recipe up to the end of Step 5, and store as directed.**

➡ When you are ready to serve this for dinner, just preheat the barbecue, then continue with the recipe from Step 6.

MEAL 2
FOR TUESDAY

ITALIAN BALSAMIC CHICKEN TRAY BAKE
(PAGE 69)

➡ **Prepare the recipe up to the end of Step 3, and store as directed.**

➡ When you are ready to serve this for dinner, simply reheat the dish as directed in Step 4.

MEAL 3
FOR WEDNESDAY

MOROCCAN TOFU AND COUSCOUS SALAD
(PAGE 70)

➡ **Prepare the recipe up to the end of Step 3, and store as directed.**

➡ When you are ready to serve this for dinner, continue with the recipe from Step 4.

Beef sausages and Thai potato salad

serves 6
preparation 45 minutes, plus cooling time,
  plus overnight chilling time
cooking 35 minutes

4 celery stalks, cut into 2 cm (¾ inch) lengths
2 carrots, cut into 2 cm (¾ inch) lengths
4 spring onions (scallions), chopped
4 eggs
1 kg (2 lb 4 oz) washed potatoes, peeled and
  cut into 1.5 cm (⅝ inch) pieces
2 tablespoons Thai spice blend (page 23)
300 g (10½ oz) light sour cream
15 g (½ oz/½ cup) coriander (cilantro) leaves
12 thin beef sausages

1 Add the celery, carrot and spring onion to the mixer bowl, measuring cup in. Chop for 5 sec/speed 7. Scrape down the side of the bowl. Chop for 3 sec/speed 5. Transfer the mixture to a large airtight container. No need to clean the mixer bowl.

2 Add 500 ml (17 fl oz/2 cups) water to the mixer bowl and insert the simmering basket. Add the eggs to the basket. Set the steaming dish on top of the mixer bowl lid. Add the potatoes to the steaming dish, making sure they are evenly spaced. Cover with the steaming dish lid. Cook for 15 min/steaming mode/speed 1.

3 Carefully remove the simmering basket with the eggs from the mixer bowl, then immediately transfer the eggs to a bowl of iced water. Peel and chop the eggs, then add them to the container with the carrot.

4 Return the steaming dish to the top of the mixer bowl with the water still inside. Stir the potatoes well, then make sure they are in an even layer in the dish. Cover with the steaming dish lid. Cook for 10 min/steaming mode/speed 1 or until just tender (you don't want them falling apart).

5 Transfer the potatoes to the container with the carrot mixture and add the spice blend, then allow to cool completely. Add the sour cream and stir to combine. Cover the airtight container, then chill overnight.

6 Preheat a barbecue chargrill plate to medium. Cook the sausages for 8–10 minutes, turning occasionally, or until cooked and golden. Serve the sausages with the potato salad.

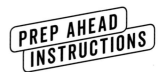

PREP AHEAD INSTRUCTIONS

The salad can be made up to 2 days ahead of serving and stored in its airtight container in the fridge.

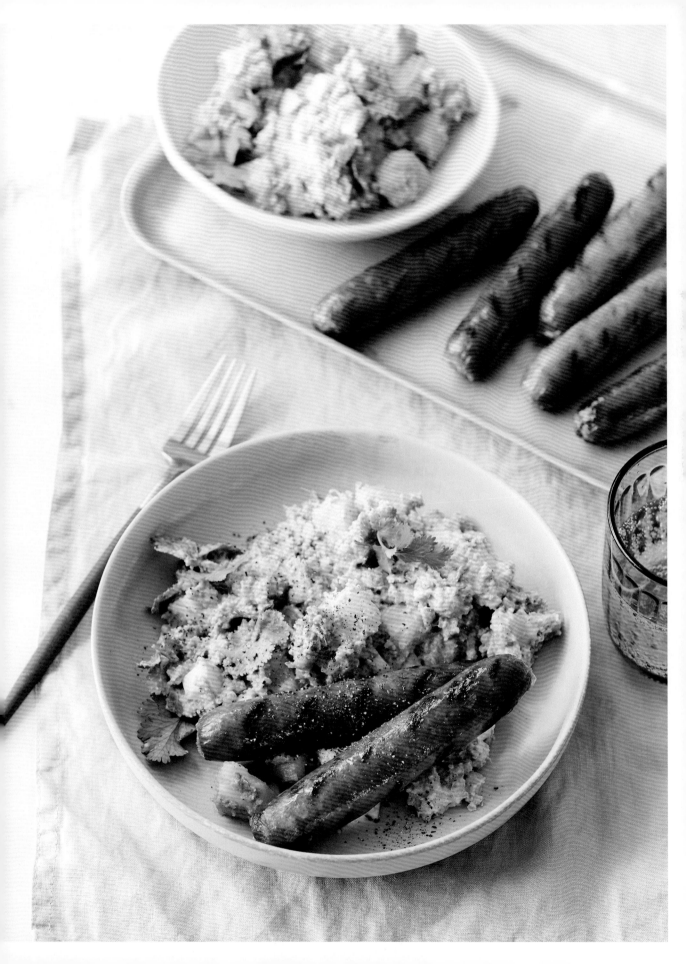

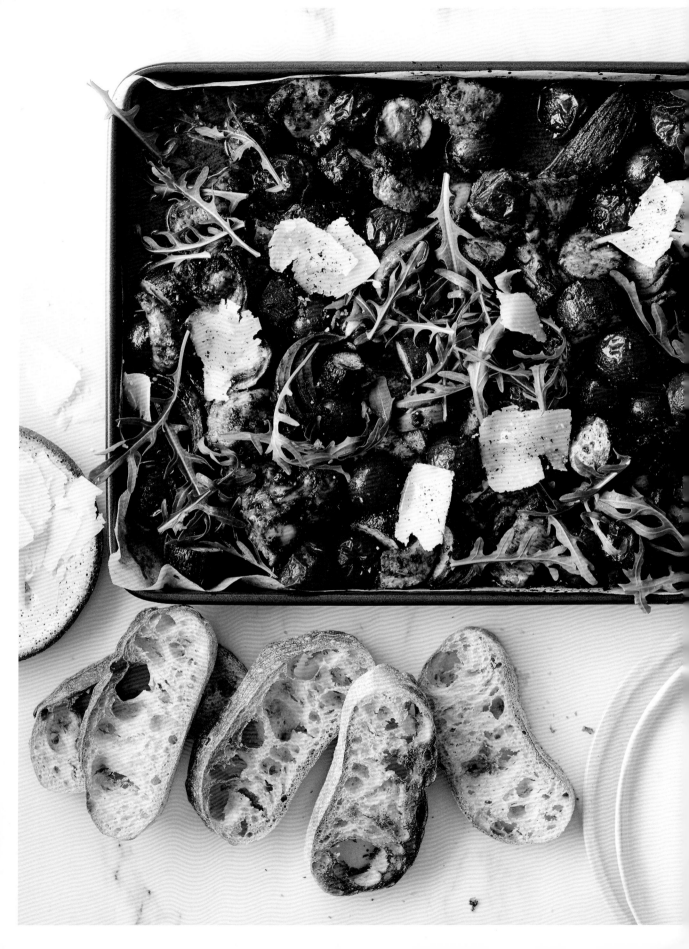

Italian balsamic chicken tray bake

serves 6
preparation 20 minutes, plus cooling time,
  plus overnight chilling time
cooking 45 minutes

1 full quantity Italian balsamic marinade (page 34)
700 g (1 lb 9 oz) diced skinless chicken breast fillets
2 red onions, cut into wedges
500 g (1 lb 2 oz) cherry tomatoes
3 zucchini (courgettes), sliced into rounds
100 g (3½ oz) baby rocket (arugula) leaves
parmesan cheese shavings, to serve
toasted ciabatta, to serve

1 Preheat the oven to 200°C (400°F)/180°C (350°F) fan-forced.
   Line a large baking tray with a small raised lip with baking paper.

2 Place the marinade, chicken, onion, tomatoes and zucchini in
   a large bowl, then toss together until well combined and evenly
   coated in the marinade.

3 Add the chicken mixture to the prepared tray, spreading it out
   in a thin layer. Bake for 25–30 minutes or until cooked and golden.
   Cool on the tray, then wrap tightly with plastic wrap and chill overnight.

4 To serve, remove the tray from the fridge while the oven preheats.
   Preheat the oven to 220°C (425°F)/200°C (400°F) fan-forced. Bake
   for 12–15 minutes or until heated through. Remove the tray from the
   oven and toss through the baby rocket. Serve straight to the table,
   sprinkled with the parmesan, and the ciabatta alongside.

Moroccan tofu and couscous salad

serves 6
preparation 20 minutes, plus 10 minutes standing time,
 plus chilling time
cooking 10 minutes

1 full quantity Moroccan marinade (page 30)
700 g (1 lb 9 oz) firm tofu, cut into 2 cm
 (¾ inch) pieces
240 g (8¾ oz/1¼ cups) couscous
375 ml (13 fl oz/1½ cups) vegetable stock
100 g (3½ oz) baby rocket (arugula) leaves
3 Lebanese (short) cucumbers, chopped
500 g (1 lb 2 oz) cherry tomatoes, halved
lemon wedges, to serve

1 Add the marinade and tofu to the mixer bowl, measuring cup in.
   Cook for 5 min/80°C/reverse stir/speed 1. Transfer to a bowl.
   No need to clean the mixer bowl.

2 Place the couscous in a separate large heatproof bowl.

3 Add the stock to the mixer bowl, measuring cup in. Heat for 3 min/
   120°C/speed 1. Transfer to the bowl with the couscous, then stir with
   a fork. Immediately cover. Stand for 10 minutes or until the couscous
   absorbs the stock. Use a fork to fluff and separate the grains. Add the
   marinated tofu. Transfer the couscous mixture to a large airtight
   container. Store in the fridge for up to 2 days.

4 Remove the couscous mixture from the fridge and add the rocket,
   cucumber and tomatoes. Toss together to combine well. Serve with
   the lemon wedges.

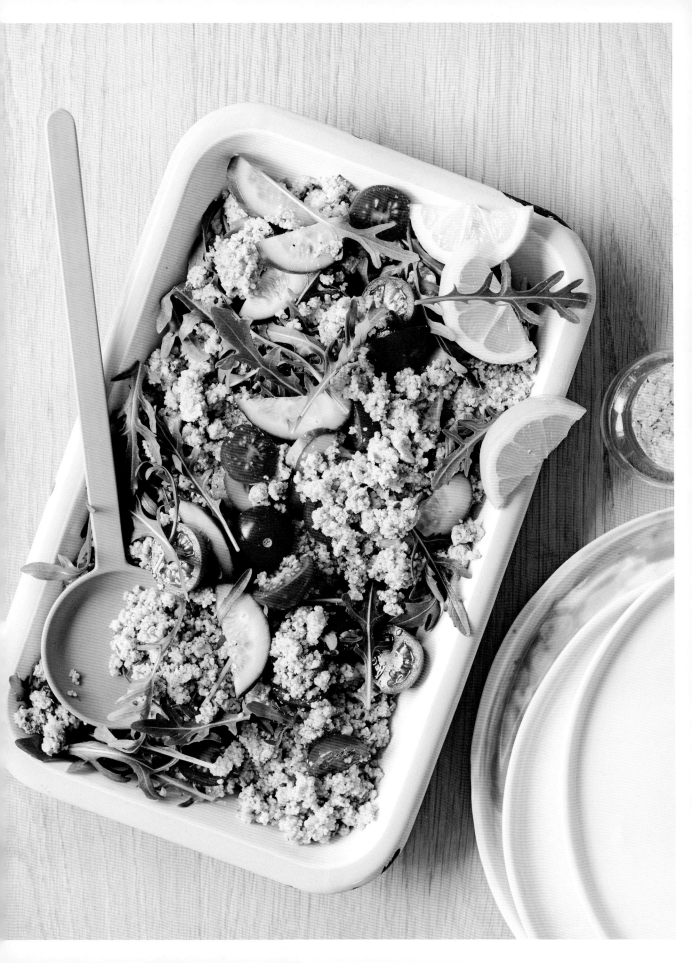

week 5

Shopping list

Fruit & veg

- [ ] 1 lime
- [ ] 1 red capsicum (pepper)
- [ ] 1 green capsicum (pepper)
- [ ] 200 g (7 oz) baby cucumbers
- [ ] 3 red onions
- [ ] 1 baby Chinese cabbage (wong bok)
- [ ] 100 g (3½ oz) snow peas (mangetout)
- [ ] 1 bunch basil
- [ ] 6 x 200 g (7 oz) baby orange sweet potatoes
- [ ] 4 spring onions (scallions)
- [ ] 1 bunch mint
- [ ] 1 bunch coriander (cilantro)
- [ ] mixed salad leaves
- [ ] 1 x 400 g (14 oz) fresh coleslaw kit

Protein

- [ ] 6 x 150 g (5½ oz) beef fillet steaks
- [ ] 12 thin chicken sausages

Pantry items

- [ ] crispy fried shallots
- [ ] 1.25 kg (2 lb 12 oz) tinned chickpeas
- [ ] 2 tablespoons avocado oil
- [ ] 6 tortillas

Fridge & freezer items

- [ ] 900 g (2 lb) thin hokkien (egg) noodles

Plus your prepped Flavour Staples

- [ ] 1 full quantity Sweet soy marinade (page 29)
- [ ] 1 full quantity Indian yoghurt marinade (page 35)
- [ ] 2 tablespoons Mexican spice blend (page 18)

Sunday prep guide

FOR MONDAY

BEEF AND OVERNIGHT NOODLES
(PAGE 74)

➡ **Prepare the recipe up to the end of Step 3, and store as directed.**

➡ When you are ready to serve this for dinner, just preheat the barbecue, then continue with the recipe from Step 4.

MEAL 2

FOR TUESDAY

INDIAN CHICKPEA-STUFFED SWEET POTATOES
(PAGE 77)

➡ **Prepare the recipe up to the end of Step 5, and store as directed.**

➡ When you are ready to serve this for dinner, simply reheat the dish as directed in Step 6.

MEAL 3

FOR WEDNESDAY

CHICKEN SAUSAGE AND COLESLAW TORTILLAS
(PAGE 78)

 Prepare the vegetables, then store them in an airtight container in the fridge.

➡ When you are ready to serve this for dinner, cook the recipe from Step 1.

Beef and overnight noodles

serves 6
preparation 25 minutes, plus cooling time,
  plus overnight chilling time
cooking 20 minutes

900 g (2 lb) thin hokkien (egg) noodles
2 red onions, cut into wedges
1 baby Chinese cabbage (wong bok), cut into wedges
1 full quantity Sweet soy marinade (page 29)
100 g (3½ oz) snow peas (mangetout), ends trimmed
6 x 150 g (5½ oz) beef fillet steaks
basil leaves, to serve
store-bought crispy fried shallots, to serve

1 Preheat a barbecue chargrill plate to high.

2 Cook the noodles in a large saucepan of boiling water according to
   the packet directions. Drain well, then transfer to a large heatproof bowl.

3 Chargrill the onion and Chinese cabbage for 10–12 minutes, turning
   occasionally, or until softened and golden. Transfer to the bowl with the
   noodles. Add the marinade, then toss well to combine. Cool completely.
   Cover tightly with plastic wrap and chill overnight.

4 Preheat a barbecue chargrill plate to high.

5 Add the snow peas to the noodle mixture and toss well to combine.
   Transfer the mixture to a large serving platter.

6 Chargrill the steaks for 3 minutes each side for medium, or cook to your
   liking. Add to the platter with the noodles. Serve sprinkled with the basil
   and crispy fried shallots.

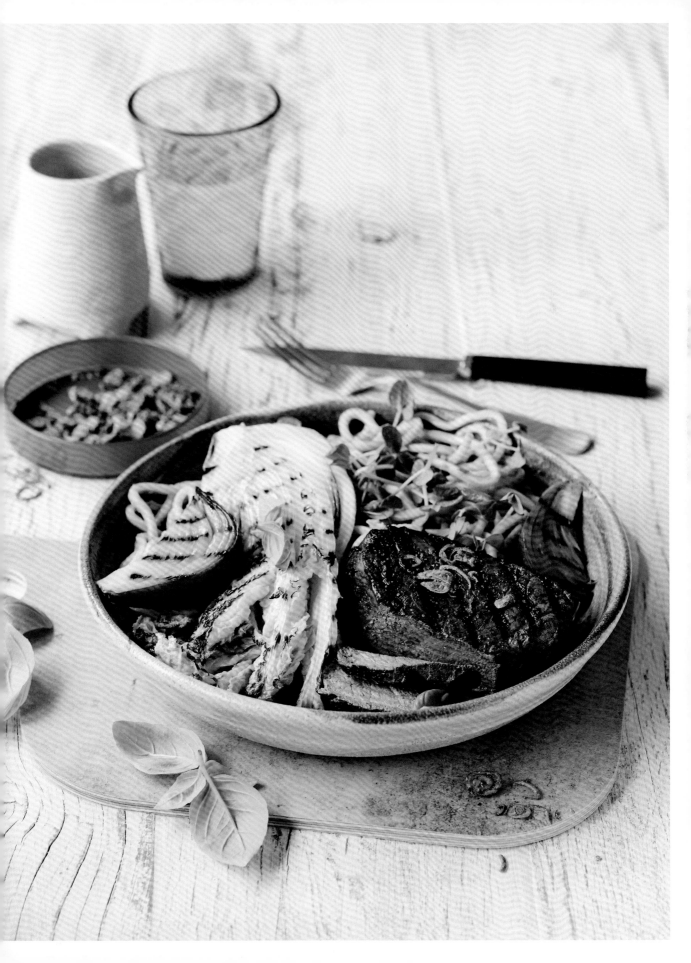

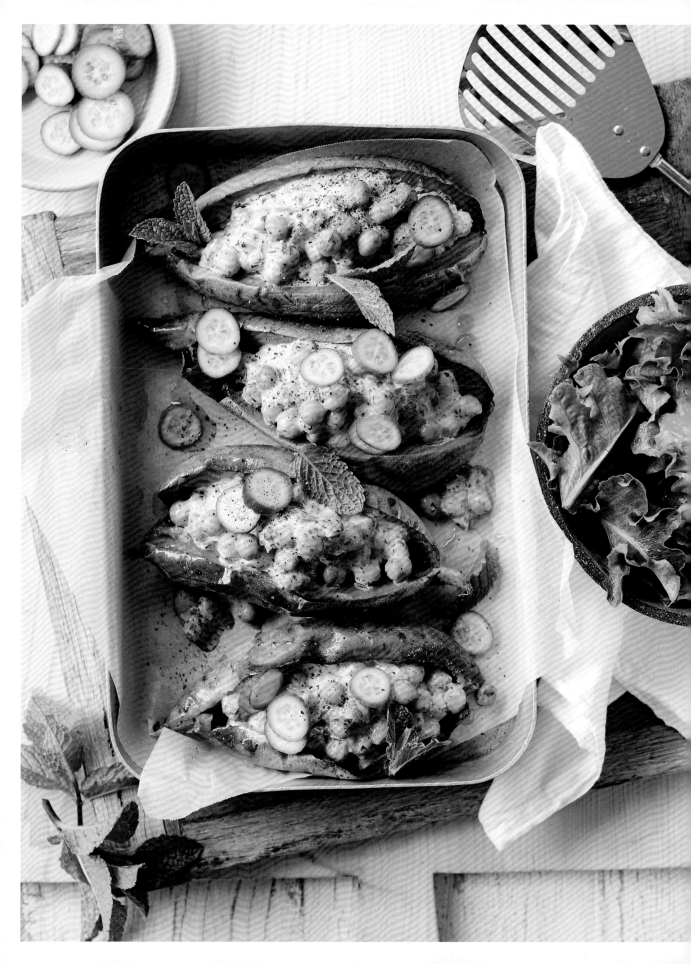

Indian chickpea-stuffed sweet potatoes

serves 6
preparation 35 minutes, plus cooling time,
  plus chilling time
cooking 1 hour 20 minutes

6 x 200 g (7 oz) baby orange sweet potatoes
4 spring onions (scallions), cut into 2 cm (¾ inch) pieces
1 full quantity Indian yoghurt marinade (page 35)
1.2 kg (2 lb 12 oz) tinned chickpeas, drained and rinsed
200 g (7 oz) baby cucumbers, thinly sliced into rounds
mint leaves, to serve
mixed salad leaves, to serve

1 Preheat the oven to 200°C (400°F)/180°C (350°F) fan-forced.

2 Place the sweet potatoes directly onto the oven shelves. Bake for
   50–60 minutes or until just tender. Remove from the oven. Cool
   completely, then transfer to a large baking dish and split each sweet
   potato lengthways down the centre, being careful not to cut all the
   way through.

3 Meanwhile, add the spring onion to the mixer bowl, measuring cup in.
   Chop for 3 sec/speed 6. Scrape down the side of the bowl. Mix for
   3 sec/speed 6.

4 Add the marinade and chickpeas to the mixer bowl, measuring cup in.
   Mix for 10 sec/reverse stir/speed 2.

5 Spoon the mixture evenly into the centre of each sweet potato in the
   baking dish. Cover the dish tightly with plastic wrap. Store in the fridge
   for up to 2 days.

6 To serve, remove the dish from the fridge while the oven preheats.
   Preheat the oven to 220°C (425°F)/200°C (400°F) fan-forced. Bake for
   20 minutes or until the sweet potatoes have heated through and crisp
   slightly around the edges. Sprinkle the tops with the cucumber and mint
   leaves. Serve the dish straight to the table with the salad alongside.

It's important to select sweet
potatoes that are the same
size in length and diameter to
ensure they cook evenly.

Chicken sausage and coleslaw tortillas

serves 6
preparation 20 minutes
cooking 10 minutes

1 red onion, quartered
2 tablespoons Mexican spice blend (page 18)
2 tablespoons avocado oil
1 red capsicum (pepper), sliced
1 green capsicum (pepper), sliced
12 thin chicken sausages
400 g (14 oz) store-bought fresh
  coleslaw salad kit, combined
6 tortillas, heated, to serve
coriander (cilantro) sprigs, to serve
lime wedges, to serve

1 Add the onion to the mixer bowl, measuring cup in. Chop for 5 sec/
   speed 7. Scrape down the side of the bowl. Chop for 5 sec/speed 7.
   Scrape down the side of the bowl.

2 Add the spice blend, oil and capsicums to the mixer bowl, measuring
   cup in. Cook for 10 min/100°C/reverse stir/speed 1.

3 Meanwhile, cook the sausages in a large, non-stick frying pan over
   medium–high heat for 8–10 minutes or until cooked and golden.

4 To serve, divide the coleslaw mixture among the heated tortillas,
   then top with the sausages and the capsicum mixture. Sprinkle with
   coriander and serve lime wedges alongside.

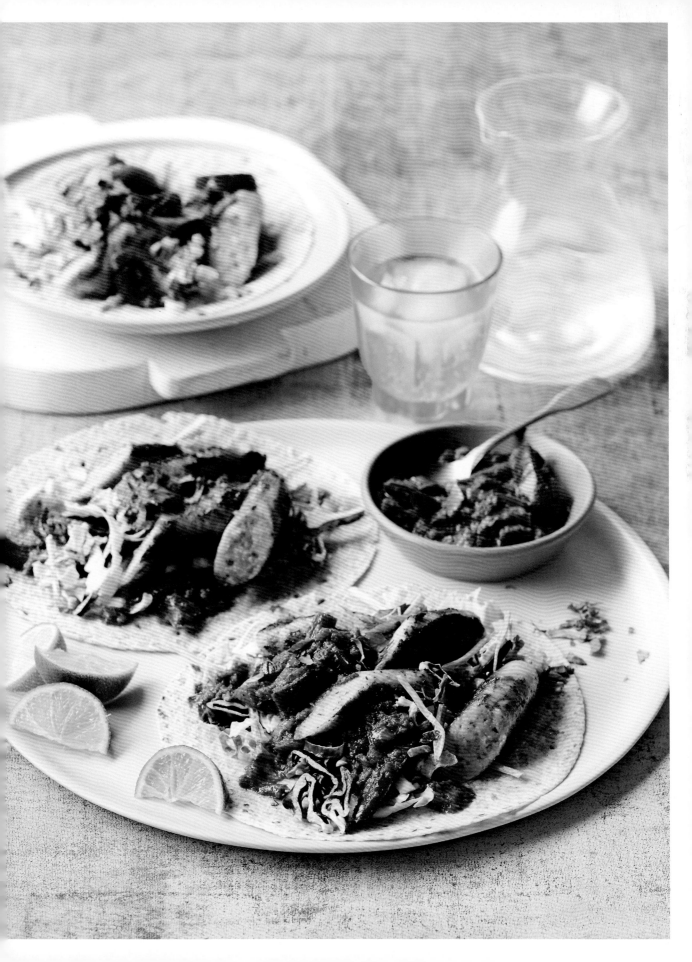

week 6

Shopping list

Fruit & veg

- [ ] 2 oranges
- [ ] 1 bunch flat-leaf (Italian) parsley
- [ ] 1 iceberg lettuce
- [ ] 1 green oakleaf lettuce
- [ ] 1 bunch baby red radishes
- [ ] 400 g (14 oz) fresh chopped vegetable mix (such as carrot, celery, leek, turnip, parsnip, broccoli, cauliflower, parsley)
- [ ] 5 cm (2 inch) piece fresh ginger
- [ ] 375 g (13 oz) fresh stir-fry vegetable mix (such as beetroot/beet, carrot, red and white cabbage, red onion, baby spinach/English spinach)

Protein

- [ ] 700 g (1 lb 9 oz) skinless flathead (or whiting) fillets
- [ ] 700 g (1 lb 9 oz) firm tofu

Pantry items

- [ ] 2 tablespoons olive oil
- [ ] 1.5 litres (52 fl oz/6 cups) vegetable stock
- [ ] 1.25 kg (2 lb 12 oz) tinned cannellini beans
- [ ] Italian croutons
- [ ] 2 tablespoons macadamia oil
- [ ] 2 tablespoons soy sauce
- [ ] 880 g (1 lb 15 oz) shelf-ready thin egg noodles

Fridge & freezer items

- [ ] 50 g (1¾ oz) butter
- [ ] garlic bread
- [ ] basil pesto

Plus your prepped Flavour Staples

- [ ] 1 tablespoon French spice blend (page 21)
- [ ] 1 full quantity Classic French marinade (page 37)
- [ ] 2 tablespoons Italian spice blend (page 14)
- [ ] 1½ tablespoons Chinese spice blend (page 24)

Sunday prep guide

MEAL 1

FOR MONDAY

FLATHEAD BISTRO SALAD WITH ORANGE
(PAGE 82)

 Prepare the recipe up to the end of Step 2, and store as directed.

 When you are ready to serve this for dinner, continue with recipe from Step 3.

MEAL 2

FOR TUESDAY

BEAN MINESTRONE
(PAGE 85)

 Prepare the recipe up to the end of Step 3, and store as directed.

 When you are ready to serve this for dinner, simply reheat the dish as directed in Step 4.

MEAL 3

FOR WEDNESDAY

CHINESE TOFU AND EGG NOODLES
(PAGE 86)

 Prepare the ginger and tofu, then store in separate airtight containers in the fridge.

 When you are ready to serve this for dinner, cook the recipe from Step 1.

Flathead bistro salad with orange

serves 6
preparation 40 minutes, plus overnight chilling time
cooking 20 minutes

1 small bunch flat-leaf (Italian) parsley,
  leaves picked
1 tablespoon French spice blend (page 21)
700 g (1 lb 9 oz) skinless flathead
  (or whiting) fillets
1 full quantity Classic French marinade (page 37)
2 oranges, skin and white pith removed,
  thinly sliced into rounds
1 iceberg lettuce, cored and cut into thin wedges
1 green oakleaf lettuce, leaves separated
1 bunch baby red radishes, very thinly
  sliced into rounds
50 g (1¾ oz) butter
garlic bread, to serve

1   Add the parsley to the mixer bowl, measuring cup in. Chop for 3 sec/
    speed 5. Scrape down the side of the bowl. Chop for 3 sec/speed 5.

2   Transfer to a large plate, add the spice blend and mix together to
    combine. Roll the flathead in the mixture to coat on all sides. Cover
    the plate tightly with plastic wrap. Chill in the fridge overnight.

3   Place the marinade, orange slices, lettuces and radish in a large bowl,
    tossing well to combine. Transfer to a large serving platter.

4   Heat a large non-stick frying pan over medium–high heat. Add half
    the butter, swirl the pan until it melts, then add half the coated flathead
    fillets. Cook for 5 minutes, then turn and cook for 5 minutes more or
    until light golden and cooked through. Transfer to the platter with the
    salad. Repeat the process once more with the remaining butter and
    remaining coated flathead fillets.

5   Serve immediately with the garlic bread alongside.

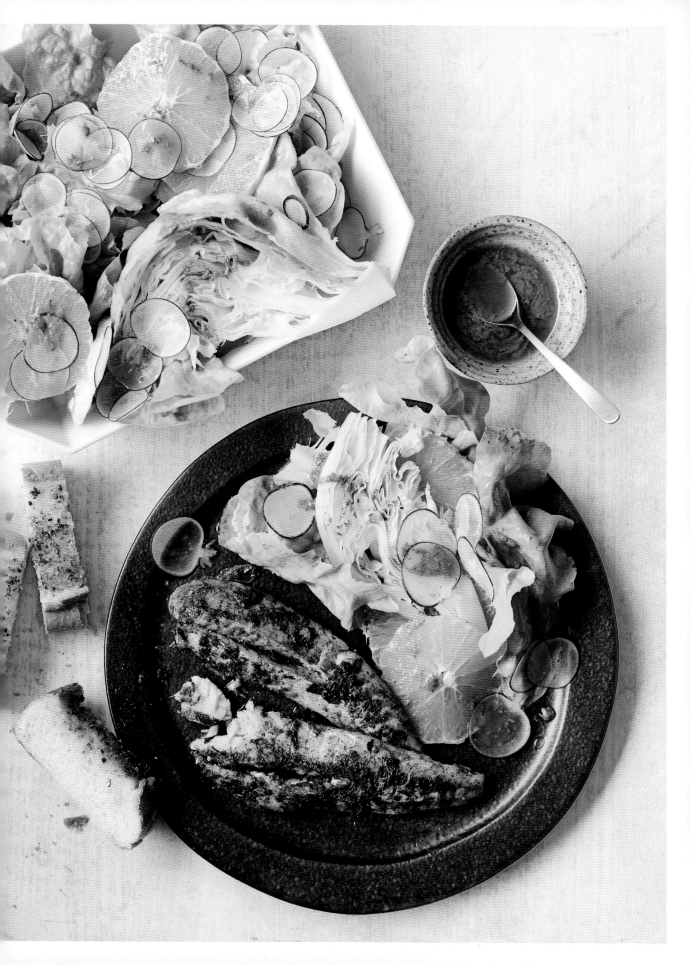

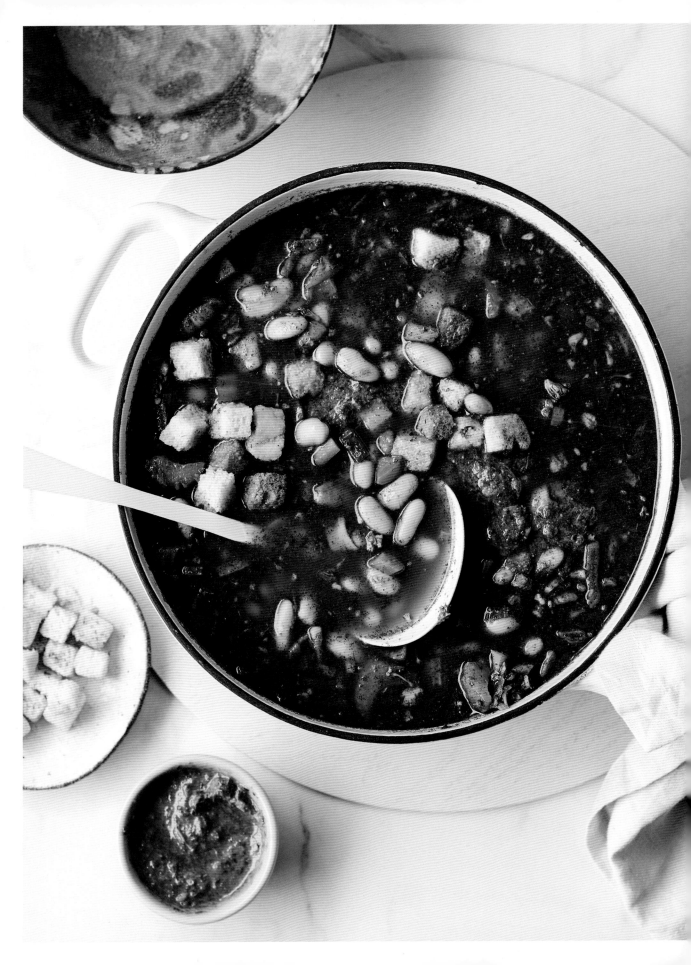

Bean minestrone

serves 6
preparation 20 minutes, plus cooling time,
  plus chilling time
cooking 20 minutes

2 tablespoons olive oil
2 tablespoons Italian spice blend (page 14)
400 g (14 oz) store-bought fresh chopped
  vegetable mix (such as carrot, celery, leek,
  turnip, parsnip, broccoli, cauliflower, parsley)
1.5 litres (52 fl oz/6 cups) vegetable stock
1.2 kg (2 lb 12 oz) tinned cannellini beans,
  drained and rinsed
store-bought Italian croutons, to serve
basil pesto, to serve

1 Add the oil, spice blend and vegetable mix to the mixer bowl,
   measuring cup in. Cook for 2 min/120°C/reverse stir/speed 1.

2 Add half the stock to the mixer bowl, measuring cup in. Cook for
   5 min/100°C/reverse stir/speed 1.

3 Add the beans to the mixer bowl, measuring cup in. Stir for 20 sec/
   reverse stir/speed 1. Transfer to an airtight container, then add the
   remaining stock. Cool completely. Store in the fridge for up to 2 days.

4 To serve, transfer the minestrone to a large saucepan and cook
   over medium–low heat, stirring occasionally, for 8–10 minutes or
   until heated through. Top with the croutons and a dollop of pesto.

Chinese tofu and egg noodles

serves 6
preparation 20 minutes, plus 3 minutes standing time
cooking 20 minutes

5 cm (2 inch) piece fresh ginger, peeled and halved
2 tablespoons macadamia oil
2 tablespoons soy sauce
1½ tablespoons Chinese spice blend (page 24)
700 g (1 lb 9 oz) firm tofu, cut into 2 cm
  (¾ inch) pieces
880 g (1 lb 15 oz) shelf-ready thin egg noodles
375 g (13 oz) store-bought fresh stir-fry vegetable mix
  (such as beetroot/beet, carrot, red and white
  cabbage, baby spinach/English spinach, red onion)

1 Add the ginger to the mixer bowl, measuring cup in. Chop for 10 sec/ speed 7. Scrape down the side of the bowl.

2 Add the oil, soy sauce and spice blend to the mixer bowl, measuring cup in. Mix for 3 sec/speed 4. Transfer the mixture to a bowl. Add the tofu. Stir well to combine and coat evenly in the spice blend mixture.

3 Heat a large non-stick wok over high heat.

4 Place the noodles in a large bowl of boiling water. Stand for 3 minutes, then drain and transfer to a large heatproof bowl.

5 Stir-fry the tofu mixture in the wok, in four batches, for 2–3 minutes each or until just cooked and golden. Transfer to the bowl with the noodles.

6 Add the vegetables to the wok, along with 60 ml (2 fl oz/¼ cup) water, and stir-fry for 2 minutes or until tender and the water has reduced by half. Return the noodles and tofu to the wok, tossing well to coat. Serve.

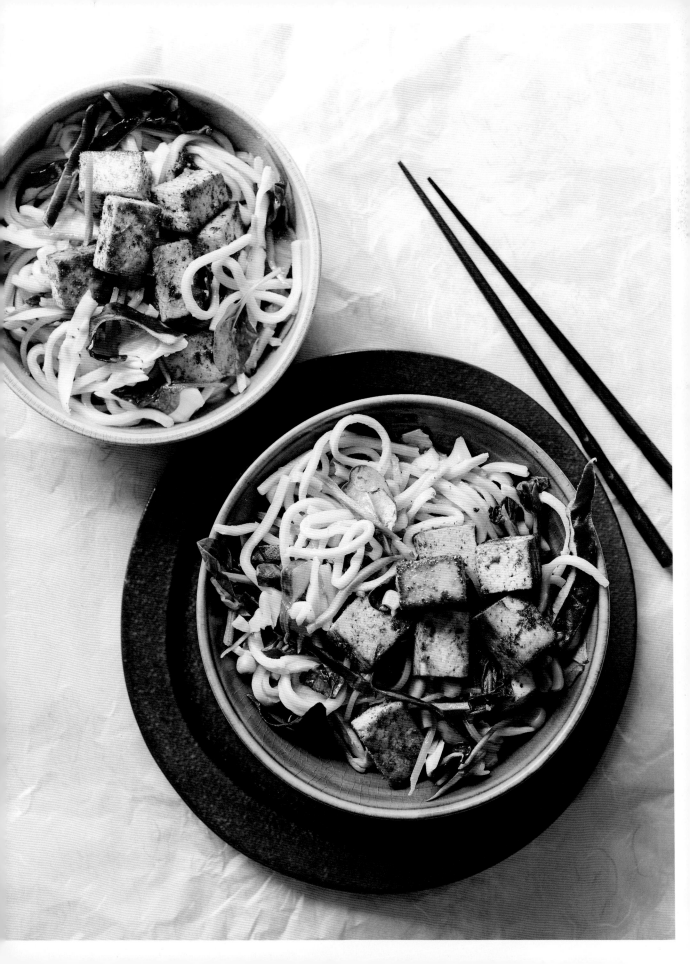

week 7

Shopping list

Fruit & veg

- ☐ 1 lime
- ☐ 1 lemon
- ☐ 500 g (1 lb 2 oz) small cherry tomatoes
- ☐ 1 large red capsicum (pepper)
- ☐ 3 zucchini (courgettes)
- ☐ 4 baby (pattypan) squash
- ☐ 2 baby cos (romaine) lettuces
- ☐ 1 leek
- ☐ 100 g (3½ oz) baby spinach (English spinach) leaves
- ☐ 2 bundles (6 pieces) baby bok choy (pak choy)
- ☐ 210 g (7½ oz/2 cups) mung bean sprouts
- ☐ 1 bunch coriander (cilantro)

Protein

- ☐ 700 g (1 lb 9 oz) beef stir-fry strips
- ☐ 700 g (1 lb 9 oz) minced (ground) chicken

Pantry items

- ☐ olive oil cooking spray
- ☐ 1 large pide (Turkish/flat bread)
- ☐ 850 g (1 lb 14 oz) tinned tuna in springwater
- ☐ 2 tablespoons olive oil
- ☐ 375 g (13 oz) dried rice-stick noodles
- ☐ toasted peanuts

Fridge & freezer items

- ☐ 630 g (1 lb 6 oz) store-bought fresh mushroom and ricotta ravioli
- ☐ 250 ml (9 fl oz/1 cup) cream for cooking

Plus your prepped Flavour Staples

- ☐ 1 full quantity Everyday mustard marinade (page 33)
- ☐ 2 tablespoons Italian spice blend (page 14)
- ☐ 1 full quantity Thai spiced marinade (page 26)

Sunday prep guide

FOR MONDAY

EVERYDAY BEEF AND VEGIE SKEWERS
(PAGE 90)

➡ Prepare the recipe up to the end of Step 2, and store as directed.

➡ When you are ready to serve this for dinner, preheat the barbecue and continue with recipe from Step 3.

MEAL 2

FOR TUESDAY

CREAMY TUNA RAVIOLI
(PAGE 93)

➡ Prepare the recipe up to the end of Step 4, and store as directed.

➡ When you are ready to serve this for dinner, simply reheat the dish as directed in Step 5.

MEAL 3

FOR WEDNESDAY

WARM THAI CHICKEN AND RICE NOODLE SALAD
(PAGE 94)

➡ Prepare the vegetables, then store them in an airtight container in the fridge.

➡ When you are ready to serve this for dinner, cook the recipe from Step 1.

Everyday beef and vegie skewers

serves 6
preparation 50 minutes, plus overnight chilling time
cooking 15 minutes

1 full quantity Everyday mustard marinade
  (page 33)
700 g (1 lb 9 oz) beef stir-fry strips
500 g (1 lb 2 oz) small cherry tomatoes
4 baby (pattypan) squash, each cut into 8 wedges
olive oil cooking spray
2 baby cos (romaine) lettuces, leaves separated
1 large pide (Turkish/flat bread), cut into 6 pieces,
  then split in half and toasted
lemon wedges, to serve

1 Combine the marinade and beef together in a large bowl. Mix well
   to coat the meat.

2 Using 18 large metal skewers, thread the coated beef strips, tomatoes
   and squash on the skewers, alternating as you go. Transfer the skewers
   to a large baking tray lined with baking paper. Cover tightly with plastic
   wrap and chill overnight.

3 Preheat a large barbecue chargrill plate to medium–high. Spray
   the skewers on all sides with oil. Cook for 10–12 minutes, turning
   occasionally, or until cooked and golden. Transfer the skewers to a
   large serving platter. Place the lettuce leaves alongside. Serve with
   the toasted pide and lemon wedges.

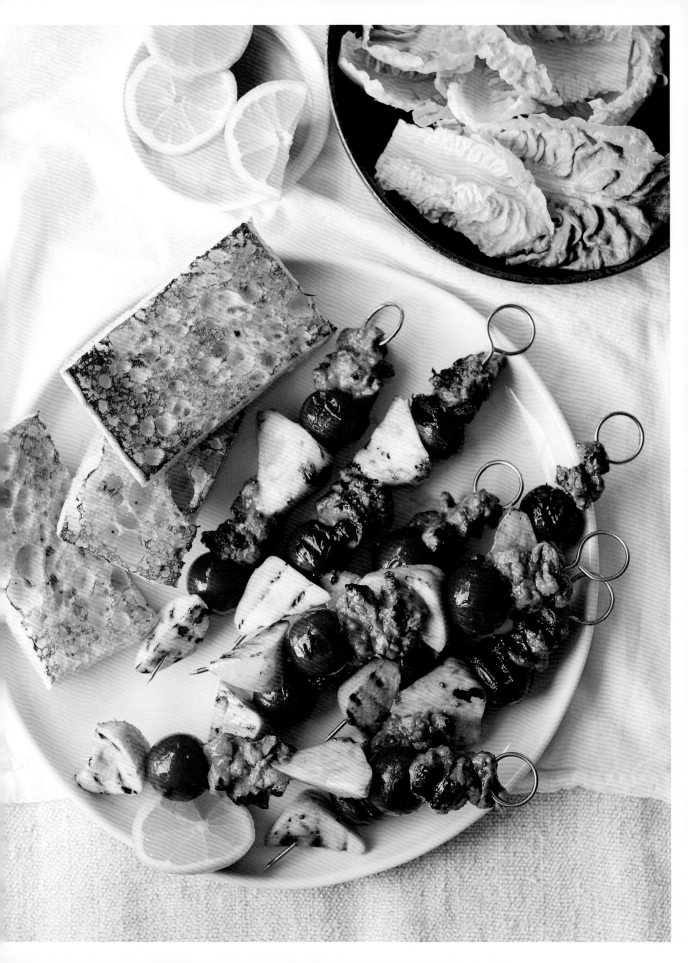

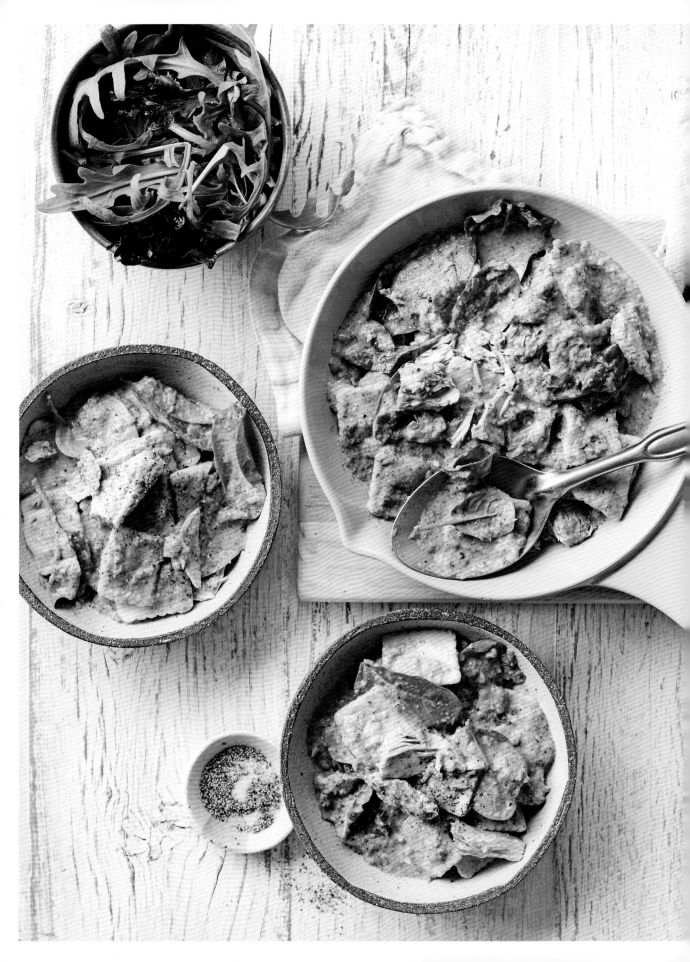

Creamy tuna ravioli

serves 6
preparation 30 minutes, plus cooling time,
  plus overnight chilling time
cooking 30 minutes

630 g (1 lb 6 oz) store-bought fresh mushroom and ricotta ravioli
850 g (1 lb 14 oz) tinned tuna in springwater, drained
1 leek, white part only, cut into 2 cm (¾ inch) pieces
3 zucchini (courgettes), cut into 2 cm (¾ inch) pieces
2 tablespoons olive oil
2 tablespoons Italian spice blend (page 14)
250 ml (9 fl oz/1 cup) cream for cooking
100 g (3½ oz) baby spinach (English spinach) leaves

1 Cook the ravioli in a large saucepan of boiling water according to
   the packet directions, minus 2 minutes' cooking time (the ravioli will
   continue to cook when reheated). Drain, reserving 500 ml (17 fl oz/
   2 cups) of the cooking water. Place the ravioli in a large heatproof bowl.
   Add the tuna, then cool completely. Store the reserved cooking water
   in a separate airtight container in the fridge overnight.

2 Add the leek and zucchini to the mixer bowl, measuring cup in. Chop
   for 5 sec/speed 7. Scrape down the side of the bowl. Chop for 5 sec/
   speed 7.

3 Add the oil and spice blend to the mixer bowl, measuring cup in.
   Cook for 10 min/100°C/speed 1 until softened. Scrape down the side
   of the bowl.

4 Add the cream to the mixer bowl, measuring cup in. Cook for
   2 min/100°C/speed 1. Add to the ravioli in the bowl and stir to combine.
   Cool completely, then cover the bowl tightly with plastic wrap. Store in
   the fridge for up to 2 days.

5 To serve, transfer the ravioli mixture to a large, deep frying pan.
   Add half the reserved cooking water. Cook, covered and stirring
   occasionally, for 8–10 minutes, adding more of the reserved cooking
   water if needed to loosen, until heated through. Remove the pan
   from the heat and stir through the spinach until wilted. Serve.

Warm Thai chicken and rice noodle salad

serves 6
preparation 30 minutes, plus 5 minutes standing time
cooking 25 minutes

1 full quantity Thai spiced marinade (page 26)
700 g (1 lb 9 oz) minced (ground) chicken
2 bundles (6 pieces) baby bok choy (pak choy),
  leaves separated
375 g (13 oz) dried rice-stick noodles
boiling water
1 large red capsicum (pepper), cut into thin strips
210 g (7½ oz/2 cups) mung bean sprouts
toasted peanuts, to serve
coriander (cilantro) leaves, to serve
lime wedges, to serve

1 Add the marinade and chicken to the mixer bowl. Cook for 5 min/120°C/
   reverse stir/speed 1. Scrape down the side of the bowl and break up
   any large lumps of mince. Remove the measuring cup and place the
   simmering basket on top of the mixer bowl lid. Cook for 20 min/100°C/
   reverse stir/speed 1.

2 Meanwhile, place the bok choy and noodles in a large bowl. Pour
   over boiling water to cover. Stand for 5 minutes or until the noodles
   have softened and separated. Drain well, then return to the same bowl.
   Add the capsicum and sprouts. Toss well to combine.

3 Add the warm chicken mixture to the noodle mixture in the bowl. Toss
   well to combine. Serve warm, sprinkled with the peanuts and coriander
   leaves, and the lime wedges alongside.

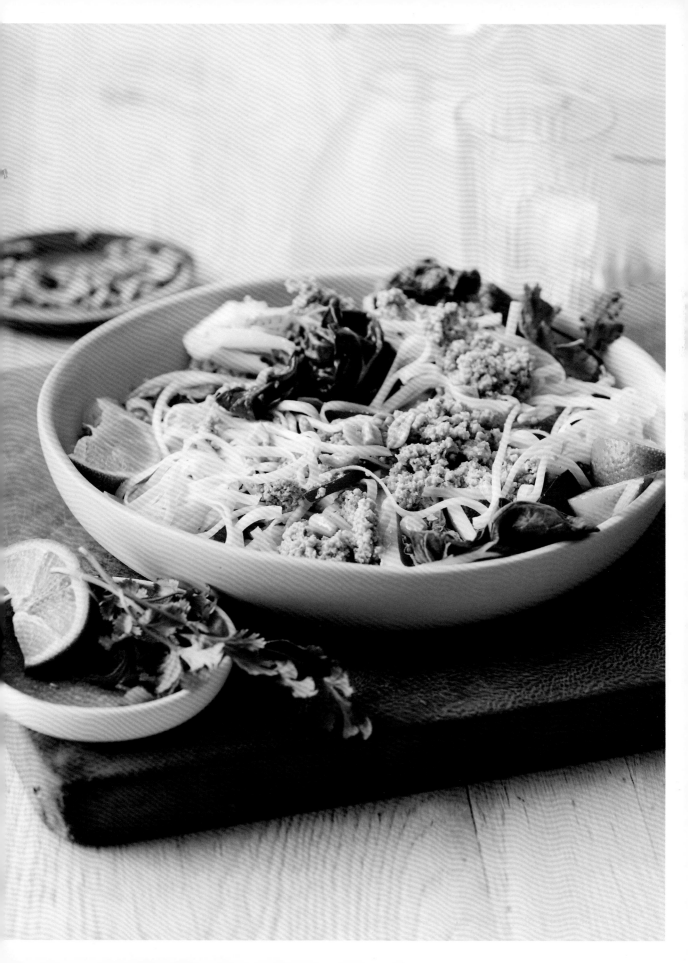

week 8

Shopping list

Fruit & veg

- [ ] 100 g (3½ oz) kale leaves
- [ ] ½ small red cabbage
- [ ] 4 spring onions (scallions)
- [ ] 1 bunch mint
- [ ] 1 onion
- [ ] 4 carrots
- [ ] 2 celery stalks
- [ ] 1 bunch basil
- [ ] mixed salad leaves

Protein

- [ ] 700 g (1 lb 9 oz) pork tenderloin

- [ ] 700 g (1 lb 9 oz) minced (ground) beef
- [ ] 1 egg

Pantry items

- [ ] 3 garlic naan
- [ ] 60 g (2¼ oz/1 cup) Japanese (panko) breadcrumbs
- [ ] olive oil cooking spray
- [ ] 800 g (1 lb 12 oz) tinned crushed tomatoes
- [ ] shelf-ready rice
- [ ] 750 g (1 lb 10 oz) dried penne pasta
- [ ] toasted pinenuts

Fridge & freezer items

- [ ] Danish feta cheese
- [ ] 500 g (1 lb 2 oz) mixed antipasto vegetables
- [ ] 220 g (7¾ oz) cherry bocconcini (fresh baby mozzarella cheese)

Plus your prepped Flavour Staples

- [ ] 1 full quantity Indian yoghurt marinade (page 35)
- [ ] 2 tablespoons Moroccan spice blend (page 25)
- [ ] 2 tablespoons Italian spice blend (page 14)

SUN DAY

Sunday prep guide

MEAL 1
FOR MONDAY

PORK NAAN
(PAGE 98)

Prepare the recipe up to the end of Step 2, and store as directed.

When you are ready to serve this for dinner, preheat the barbecue and continue with recipe from Step 3.

MEAL 2
FOR TUESDAY

MOROCCAN MEATBALL AND CHICKPEA BAKE
(PAGE 101)

Prepare the recipe up to the end of Step 5, and store as directed.

When you are ready to serve this for dinner, simply reheat the dish as directed in Step 6.

MEAL 3
FOR WEDNESDAY

ANTIPASTO PASTA
(PAGE 102)

Prepare the vegetables, then store them in an airtight container in the fridge.

When you are ready to serve this for dinner, cook the recipe from Step 1.

Pork naan

serves 6
preparation 25 minutes, plus overnight chilling time
cooking 10 minutes

100 g (3½ oz) kale leaves, torn
½ small red cabbage, cored and cut into 4
4 spring onions (scallions), sliced
20 g (¾ oz/1 cup) mint leaves
1 full quantity Indian yoghurt marinade (page 35)
700 g (1 lb 9 oz) pork tenderloin, sinew removed,
  halved lengthways and thinly sliced crossways
3 garlic naan, split in half and toasted

1 Add the kale to the mixer bowl, measuring cup in. Chop for 3 sec/
   speed 7, or until finely chopped. Transfer to a bowl.

2 Add the cabbage, spring onion and mint to the mixer bowl, measuring
   cup in. Chop for 3 sec/speed 7. Scrape down the side of the bowl.
   Chop for 3 sec/speed 4. Transfer to the bowl with the kale. Add three-
   quarters of the marinade and stir to combine well. Cover tightly with
   plastic wrap. Chill overnight.

3 Preheat a barbecue flatplate to high. Cook the pork for 8–10 minutes,
   turning occasionally, or until cooked and golden.

4 To serve, divide the cabbage mixture on top of the toasted naan,
   then top with the pork and drizzle with the remaining marinade.

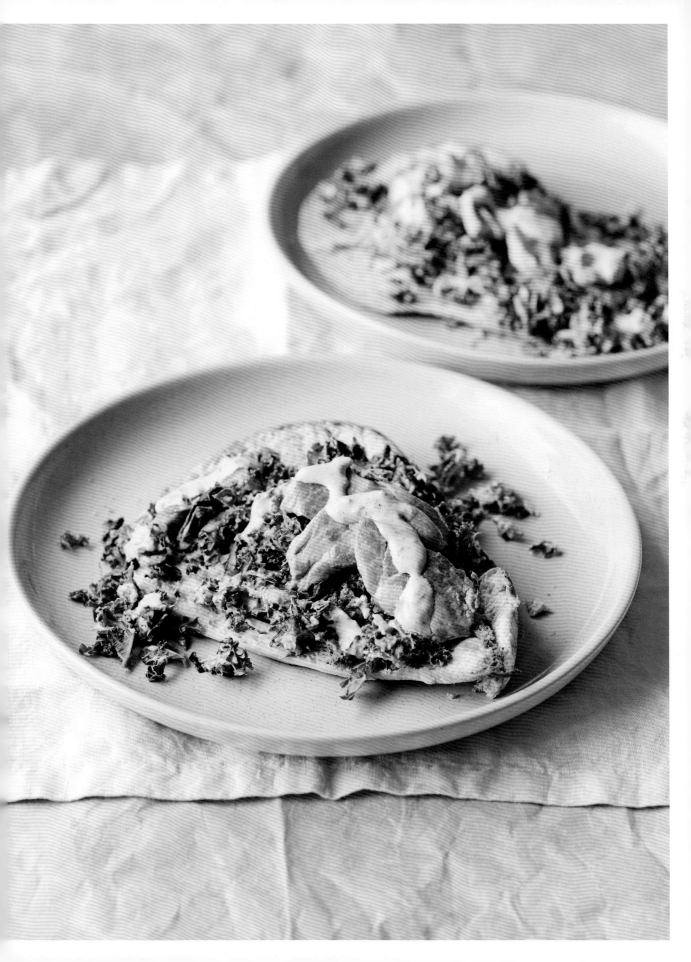

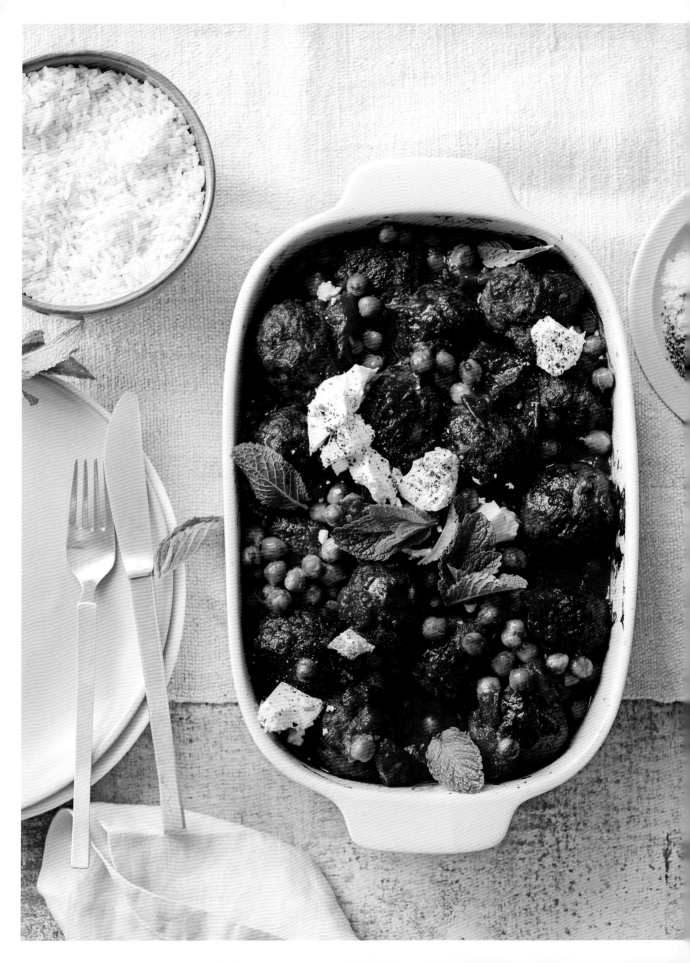

Moroccan meatball and chickpea bake

serves 6
preparation 45 minutes, plus cooling time,
 plus chilling time
cooking 40 minutes

1 onion, quartered
1 carrot, cut into 2 cm (¾ inch) pieces
1 egg
2 tablespoons Moroccan spice blend (page 25)
700 g (1 lb 9 oz) minced (ground) beef
60 g (2¼ oz/1 cup) Japanese (panko) breadcrumbs
olive oil cooking spray
800 g (1 lb 12 oz) tinned crushed tomatoes
Danish feta cheese, to serve
mint leaves, to serve
cooked rice, to serve

1 Preheat the oven to 220°C (425°F)/200°C (400°F) fan-forced.

2 Add the onion and carrot to the mixer bowl, measuring cup in. Chop
   for 5 sec/speed 7. Scrape down the side of the bowl. Chop for 5 sec/
   speed 7 or until finely chopped. Scrape down the side of the bowl.

3 Add the egg and spice blend to the mixer bowl, measuring cup in.
   Mix for 5 sec/speed 4.

4 Transfer the mixture to a large bowl. Add the beef and breadcrumbs.
   Using clean hands, mix everything together until well combined, then
   shape firmly into 18 equal-sized meatballs.

5 Transfer the meatballs to a large baking dish and spray with oil. Bake in
   the oven for 20 minutes, turning occasionally, until cooked and browned
   on all sides. Remove the dish from the oven, add the crushed tomatoes
   and stir to combine. Cool completely. Cover the dish tightly with plastic
   wrap. Store in the fridge for up to 2 days.

6 To serve, remove the dish from the fridge while the oven preheats.
   Preheat the oven to 200°C (400°F)/180°C (350°F) fan forced. Remove
   the plastic wrap. Bake for 20 minutes or until the meatballs have
   reheated and the tomatoes are bubbling. Remove from the oven and
   sprinkle the top with the feta, then the mint and serve the dish straight
   to the table with the rice alongside.

Antipasto pasta

serves 6
preparation 25 minutes
cooking 25 minutes

750 g (1 lb 10 oz) dried penne pasta
2 celery stalks, cut into 2 cm (¾ inch) pieces
3 carrots, cut into 2 cm (¾ inch) pieces
2 tablespoons Italian spice blend (page 14)
500 g (1 lb 2 oz) mixed antipasto vegetables
220 g (7¾ oz) cherry bocconcini (fresh baby
  mozzarella cheese), torn
basil leaves, to serve
toasted pine nuts, to serve
mixed salad leaves, to serve

1 Cook the pasta in a large saucepan of boiling water according to
   the packet directions. Drain well, then transfer to a large bowl.
   Cover to keep warm.

2 Meanwhile, add the celery and carrot to the mixer bowl, measuring
   cup in. Chop for 5 sec/speed 7. Scrape down the side of the bowl.
   Chop for 5 sec/speed 7. Scrape down the side of the bowl.

3 Add the spice blend to the mixer bowl, measuring cup in. Cook for
   5 min/120°C/reverse stir/speed 1.

4 Transfer the vegetable mixture to the bowl with the pasta. Add the
   antipasto vegetables, then toss well to combine. Serve topped with
   the bocconcini, basil and pine nuts, with the mixed salad alongside.

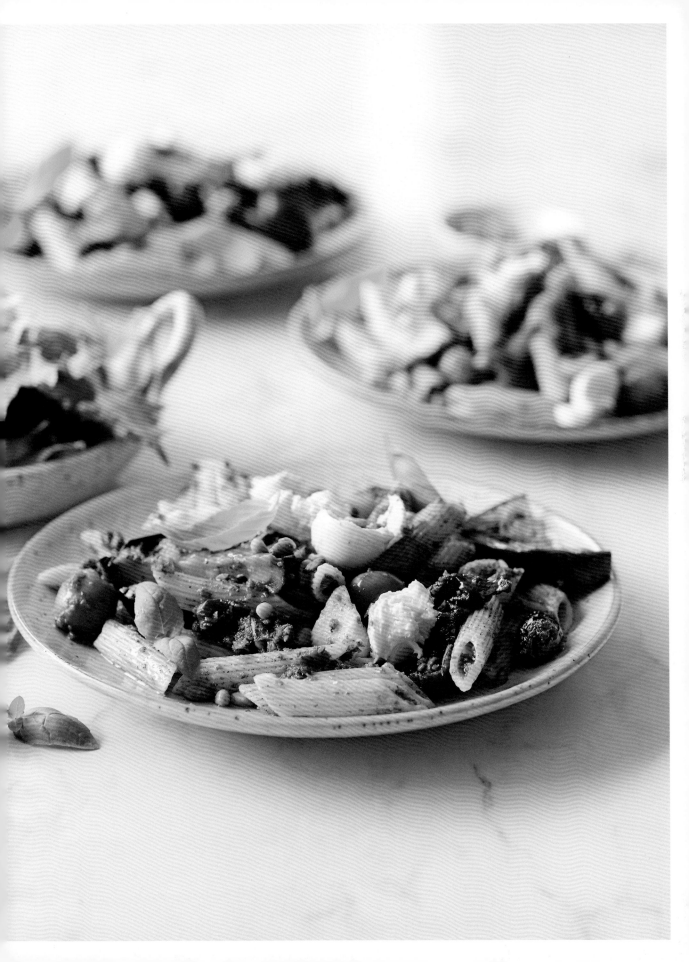

5-ingredient flavour- boosted meals

This section is filled with recipes for delicious and fresh flavour boosters, which are designed to be dolloped onto, drizzled over or served alongside meals. For each flavour booster, I have included three mini recipes. And to make life super easy, these recipes use only a maximum of five ingredients.

Again, all you need to do is prep the flavour boosters ahead of time, then store them in your fridge or freezer. As well as the mini recipes, I've also provided loads of other great ideas for how to use these flavour boosters in your cooking.

STORING FLAVOUR BOOSTERS

1 full quantity
The flavour boosters will keep in an airtight container in the fridge for up to 3 days (fresh herbs will discolour slightly).

2 full quantities
The flavour boosters will keep in two separate airtight containers in the freezer for up to 2 months. Defrost in the fridge overnight (fresh herbs will discolour slightly).

4 full quantities
The flavour boosters will keep in four separate airtight containers in the freezer for up to 2 months. Defrost in the fridge overnight (fresh herbs will discolour slightly).

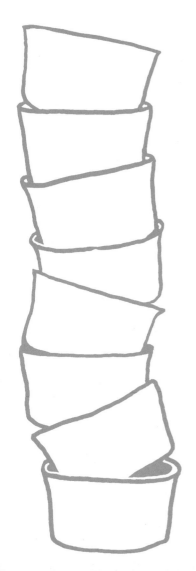
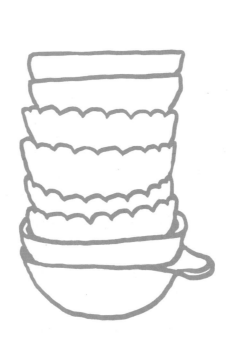
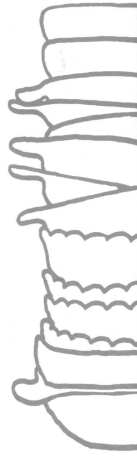

Coriander lime pesto

makes approximately 250 g (9 oz/1 cup)
preparation 15 minutes

1 small garlic clove
1 small red chilli, halved
55 g (2 oz/⅓ cup) toasted macadamia nuts
1 bunch coriander (cilantro), well washed,
  stems and leaves torn
15 g (½ oz/½ cup) basil leaves
zest and juice of 2 large limes
60 ml (2 fl oz/¼ cup) avocado oil

1 Add the garlic, chilli and macadamia nuts to the mixer bowl, measuring
   cup in. Chop for 10 sec/speed 9. Scrape down the side of the bowl.

2 Add the remaining ingredients to the mixer bowl, measuring cup in.
   Chop for 20 sec/speed 7.

TRY THIS

Add a dollop to a bowl of soup

Use as a dip for cooked prawns (shrimp)

Add to foil parcels of chopped vegies, then bake

Spoon over chargrilled fish

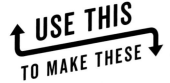

USE THIS TO MAKE THESE

Beef noodles

In a large bowl, place 1 full quantity of the **pesto**; 6 x 120 g (4¼ oz) **beef fillet steaks**, chargrilled; 250 g (9 oz) **thick rice noodles**, soaked, then drained and 300 g (10½ oz) **mixed salad leaves**. Toss everything together to combine, then serve.

Tofu noodles

In a large bowl place 1 full quantity of the **pesto**; 700 g (1 lb 9 oz) sliced **firm tofu**, chargrilled; 250 g (9 oz) **thin rice-stick noodles**, soaked, then drained; 500 g (1 lb 2 oz) **green beans**, trimmed and blanched and 500 g (1 lb 2 oz) halved **cherry tomatoes**. Toss everything together to combine, then serve.

Chicken noodles

In a large bowl place 1 full quantity of the **pesto**; 700 g (1 lb 9 oz) skinless **chicken breast fillet,** chargrilled, then sliced; 200 g (7 oz) **rice vermicelli**, soaked, then drained; 2 bundles **baby bok choy** (pak choy), leaves separated and blanched and 1 thinly sliced large **red capsicum** (pepper). Toss everything together to combine, then serve.

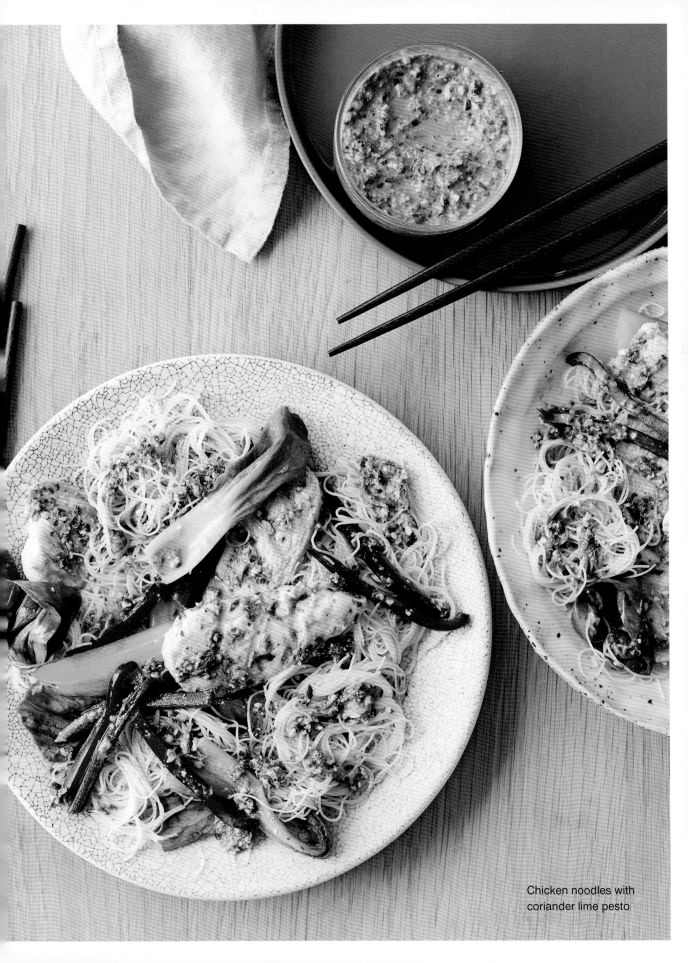

Chicken noodles with
coriander lime pesto

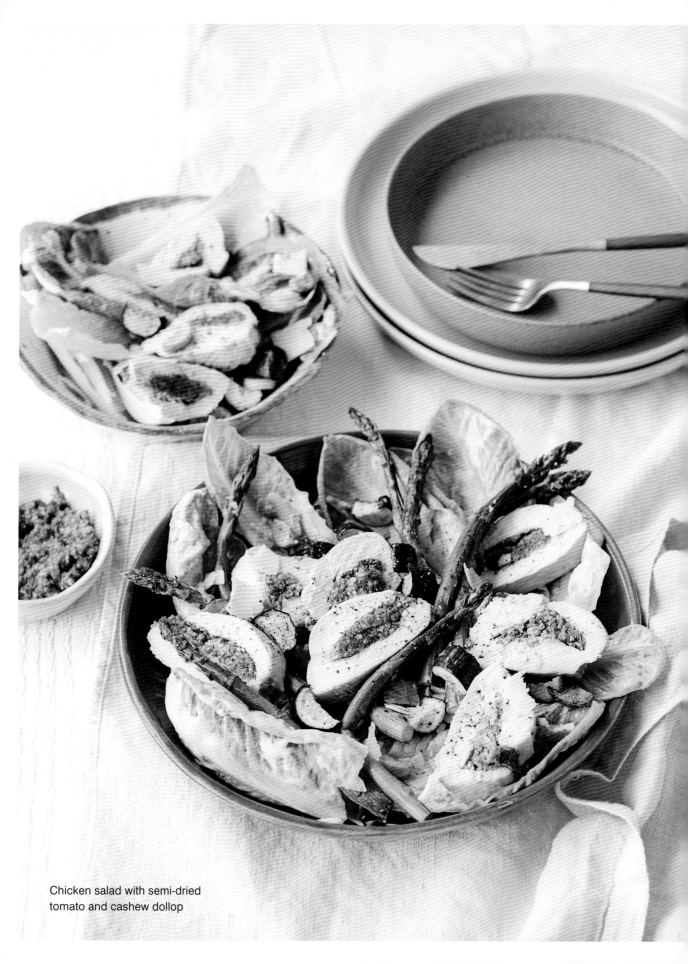

Chicken salad with semi-dried
tomato and cashew dollop

Semi-dried tomato and cashew dollop

makes approximately 450 g (1 lb/1¾ cups)
preparation 15 minutes

160 g (5½ oz/¾ cup) semi-dried (sun-blushed) tomatoes in oil
1 teaspoon Italian spice blend (page 14)
120 g (4¼ oz/¾ cup) toasted cashews
zest and juice of 1 lemon
35 g (1¼ oz/⅓ cup) finely grated parmesan cheese
80 ml (2½ fl oz/⅓ cup) extra virgin olive oil

Add the tomatoes, spice blend and cashews to the mixer bowl, measuring cup in. Chop for 10 sec/speed 9. Repeat the chopping again (scraping down the side of the bowl) until a chunky paste forms. Add the remaining ingredients to the mixer bowl. Chop for 20 sec/speed 7.

TRY THIS

Spread over layers of lasagne before baking

Serve with crudités

Add to wraps with falafel and salad leaves

Dollop over frittata mixture before cooking

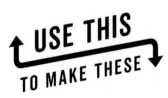

USE THIS TO MAKE THESE

Chicken salad

Preheat the oven to 220°C (425°F)/200°C (400°F) fan-forced. Line a baking tray with baking paper. Spread 1 full quantity of the **dollop** evenly over one half of 6 butterflied skinless **chicken breast fillets**, then fold up to enclose. Secure with toothpicks. Place on the tray with 4 thickly sliced **zucchini** (courgettes) and 2 trimmed bunches of **asparagus**. Roast for 25–30 minutes or until cooked. Divide a store-bought 290 g (10¼ oz) **Caesar salad kit** (with dressing and croutons) among serving plates, top with the vegetables and sliced chicken and serve.

Eggplant salad

Preheat the oven to 220°C (425°F)/200°C (400°F) fan-forced. Line a baking tray with baking paper. Spread 1 full quantity of the **dollop** evenly over the cut sides of 3 medium **eggplants** (aubergines), halved lengthways and scored. Place on the tray with 6 sliced **zucchini** (courgettes) and 2 trimmed bunches of **asparagus**. Roast for 25–30 minutes or until cooked. Divide a store-bought 290 g (10¼ oz) **Caesar salad kit** (with dressing and croutons) among serving plates, top with the vegetables and serve.

Beef salad

Preheat the oven to 220°C (425°F)/200°C (400°F) fan-forced. Line a baking tray with baking paper. Spread 1 full quantity of the **dollop** evenly over 6 (400 g/14 oz in total) **beef sizzle steaks**, then roll up and secure with toothpicks. Place on the tray with 4 sliced **zucchini** (courgettes) and 2 trimmed bunches of **asparagus**. Roast for 25–30 minutes or until cooked. Divide a store-bought 290 g (10¼ oz) **Caesar salad kit** (with dressing and croutons) among serving plates, top with the vegetables and sliced beef rolls and serve.

Chimichurri

makes approximately 160 g (5½ oz/⅔ cup)
preparation 15 minutes

1 small garlic clove
25 g (1 oz/¾ cup) coriander (cilantro) leaves
15 g (½ oz/¾ cup) flat-leaf (Italian) parsley leaves
1 teaspoon dried chilli flakes
1 teaspoon smoked paprika
60 ml (2 fl oz/¼ cup) red wine vinegar
60 ml (2 fl oz/¼ cup) avocado oil

Add all the ingredients to the mixer bowl, measuring cup in.
Chop for 20 sec/speed 7. Scrape down the side of the bowl.

TRY THIS

Toss with cut tomatoes
and serve on toast

Drizzle over fried eggs

Drizzle over tofu skewers

**Add to parcels of white
fish before baking**

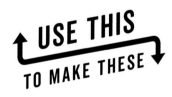

USE THIS TO MAKE THESE

Pork fajitas

Toss 1 full quantity of the
chimichurri with 700 g (1 lb 9 oz)
pork fillet, chargrilled, then sliced;
6 mixed coloured **capsicums**
(peppers), sliced, then chargrilled;
and 2 sliced **avocados**. Divide
among 12 **wholegrain tortillas**,
fold up and serve.

Prawn parcels

Toss 1 full quantity of the
chimichurri with 700 g (1 lb 9 oz)
large peeled and deveined **raw
prawns** (shrimp), chargrilled;
250 g (9 oz) store-bought **raw
zucchini (courgette) spaghetti**
and 2 chopped **avocados**. Divide
among 18 small **iceberg lettuce**
cups and serve.

Lamb wraps

Take 1 full quantity of the
chimichurri and toss half of it over
700 g (1 lb 9 oz) **lamb backstrap**
(loin fillet), chargrilled, then sliced;
200 g (7 oz) **mixed salad leaves**
and 2 sliced **avocados**. Divide
among 6 **wholegrain soft wraps**,
drizzle with the remaining
chimichurri, roll up and serve.

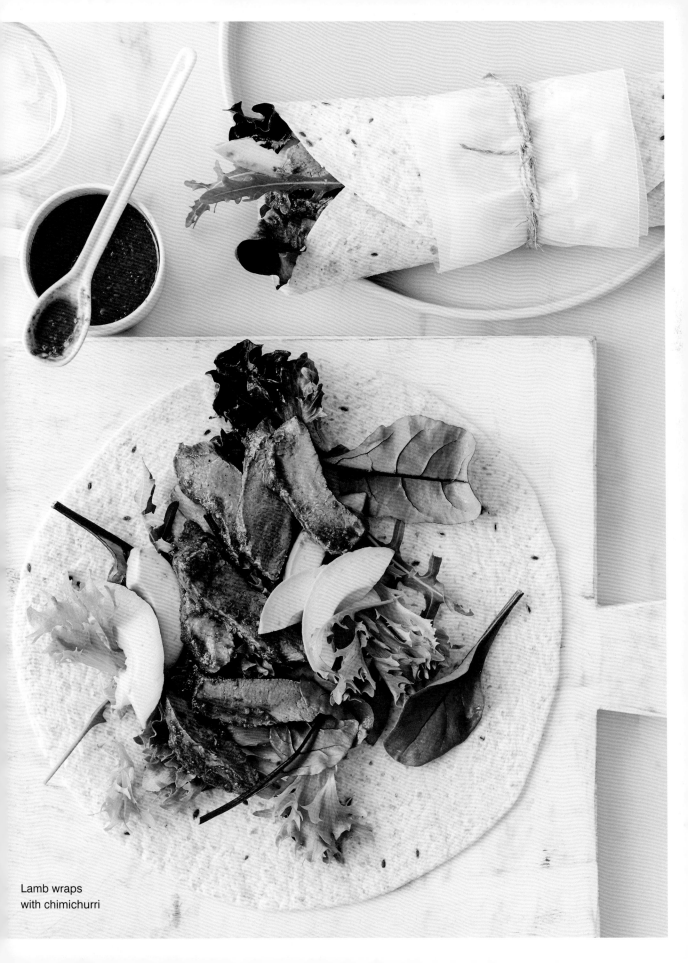

Lamb wraps
with chimichurri

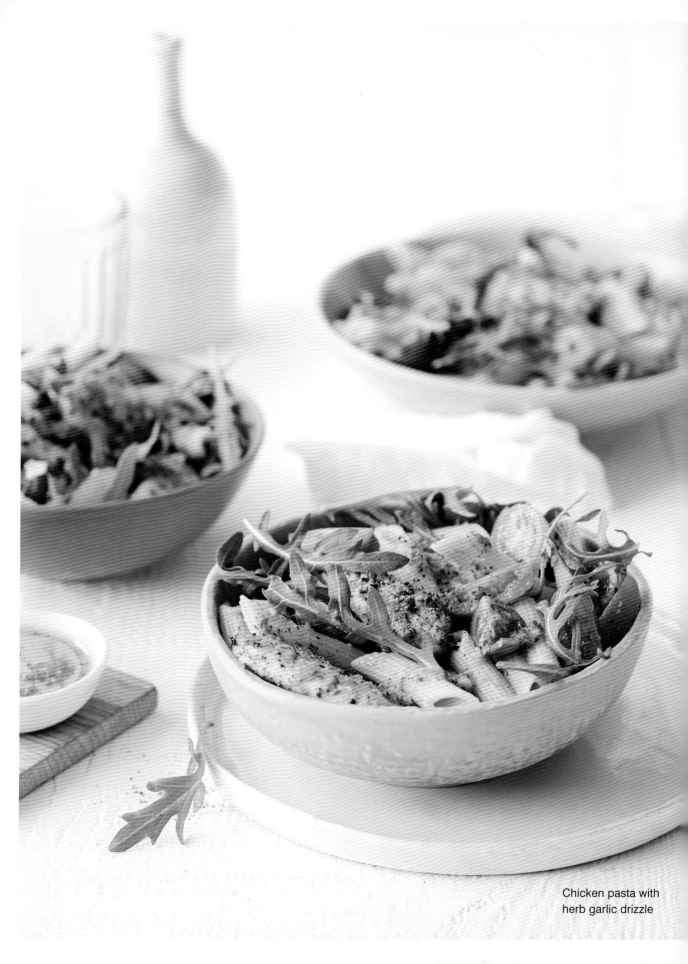

Chicken pasta with
herb garlic drizzle

Herb garlic drizzle

makes approximately 155 g (5½ oz/¾ cup)
preparation 15 minutes

10 garlic cloves
125 ml (4 fl oz/½ cup) olive oil
1 teaspoon sea salt
¼ teaspoon white sugar

2 tablespoons oregano
leaves, chopped
2 tablespoons finely chopped
chives

1 Add the garlic to the mixer bowl, measuring cup in. Chop for 5 sec/
speed 9 and repeat the chopping (scraping down the side of the bowl
each time) until a paste forms.

2 Remove the measuring cup. Mix for 2 min/speed 4, while slowly pouring
in the oil until completely blended.

3 Add the remaining ingredients. Stir for 10 sec/reverse stir/speed 4 until
well combined.

STORAGE

The drizzle will keep in an
airtight container in the fridge
for up to 7 days (fresh herbs
will discolour slightly).

TRY THIS

Spread over mini pitta breads
– add tabouleh and lemon

Use as a dip for meatballs

Stir with mayo to make aïoli

**Use as base for any vegie
soup mixture**

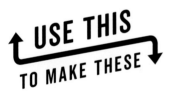

USE THIS TO MAKE THESE

Chicken pasta

Preheat a grill (broiler) to high.
Line a baking tray with foil. Toss
together 1 full quantity of the
drizzle and 700 g (1 lb 9 oz)
chicken tenderloins, halved
diagonally. Add to the tray. Grill for
8–10 minutes, turning occasionally,
until cooked and golden. Transfer
to a heatproof bowl. Add 600 g
(1 lb 5 oz) quartered **medley baby
tomatoes**, 100 g (3½ oz) **baby
rocket** (arugula) leaves and 750 g
(1 lb 10 oz) cooked **penne pasta**.
Toss well, then serve.

Tomato pasta

Preheat a grill (broiler) to high. Line
a baking tray with foil. Spread 1 full
quantity of the **drizzle** evenly over
8 halved **vine-ripened tomatoes**.
Add to the tray with 4 bunches of
asparagus, trimmed and halved.
Grill for 10–15 minutes, turning the
asparagus only occasionally, until
cooked and golden. Transfer to a
heatproof bowl. Add 2 chopped
avocados and 750 g (1 lb 10 oz)
cooked **fusilli pasta**. Toss well,
then serve.

Salmon pasta

Preheat a grill (broiler) to high.
Line a baking tray with foil. Spread
1 full quantity of the **drizzle** evenly
over the tops of 6 x 120 g (4¼ oz)
skinless, boneless **salmon
portions**. Add to the tray. Grill for
10–15 minutes, until cooked and
the tops are golden. Transfer to
a heatproof bowl. Add 600 g
(1 lb 5 oz) quartered **medley baby
tomatoes**, 100 g (3½ oz) **baby
rocket** (arugula) leaves and 750 g
(1 lb 10 oz) cooked **spaghetti**. Toss
well, breaking up the salmon into
large pieces, then serve.

Sweet chilli sauce

makes approximately 350 g (12 oz/1½ cups)
preparation 15 minutes
cooking 30 minutes

1 garlic clove
3 cm (1¼ inch) piece fresh
  ginger, peeled
6 long red chillies, cut into 4
2 red onions, quartered

185 g (6½ oz/1 cup) brown
  sugar
60 ml (2 fl oz/¼ cup) white
  vinegar
2 teaspoons fish sauce

1 Place the garlic, ginger, chillies and onion in the mixer bowl, measuring
   cup in. Chop for 10 sec/speed 7. Scrape down the side of the bowl.
   Chop for 10 sec/speed 7. Scrape down the side of the bowl.

2 Add the remaining ingredients to the mixer bowl, measuring cup in.
   Cook for 30 min/100°C/speed 1.5 or until the mixture is slightly
   thickened. Use as required or cool completely before storing.

STORAGE

The sauce will keep in an
airtight container in the fridge
for up to 7 days.

TRY THIS

Use to marinate beef steaks
before barbecuing

Add to mashed sweet potato

Mix with spreadable cream
cheese for a dip or sandwich
spread

**Serve with sour cream
and potato wedges**

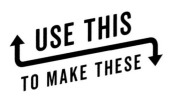

USE THIS TO MAKE THESE

Sticky pork and rice

Preheat a barbecue flatplate to
medium. Coat 700 g (1 lb 9 oz)
pork stir-fry strips in 1 full
quantity of the **sauce**. Cook on
the barbecue for 10–12 minutes,
turning occasionally, or until
cooked and caramelised.
Transfer to a large heatproof bowl.
Add 500 g (1 lb 2 oz) store-bought
fresh shredded **coleslaw mix**
and 500 g (1 lb 2 oz) cooked and
heated shelf-ready **basmati
coconut rice**. Toss together until
well combined. Serve with **lime
wedges** squeezed over.

Sticky chicken and rice

Preheat a barbecue flatplate to
medium. Coat 700 g (1 lb 9 oz)
chicken tenderloins in 1 full
quantity of the **sauce**. Cook on
the barbecue for 12–15 minutes,
turning occasionally, or until
cooked and caramelised. Transfer
to a large heatproof bowl. Add
4 sliced **zucchini** (courgettes)
to the barbecue. Cook, tossing,
for 5 minutes or until just cooked.
Add to the bowl with the chicken.
Add 500 g (1 lb 2 oz) cooked and
heated shelf-ready **basmati
coconut rice**. Toss together until
well combined. Serve with **lemon
wedges** squeezed over.

Sticky salmon and rice

Preheat a barbecue flatplate to low.
Coat 6 x 120 g (4¼ oz) skinless,
boneless **salmon portions** in 1 full
quantity of the **sauce**. Barbecue for
8 minutes, turning occasionally,
for medium, or cook to your liking.
Transfer to a large heatproof bowl.
Add 500 g (1 lb 2 oz) trimmed **snow
peas** (mangetout) to the barbecue.
Cook, tossing, for 2 minutes or until
just cooked. Add to the bowl with
the salmon. Add 500 g (1 lb 2 oz)
cooked and heated shelf-ready
basmati coconut rice. Toss until
combined and the salmon breaks
up into large pieces. Serve with
lime wedges squeezed over.

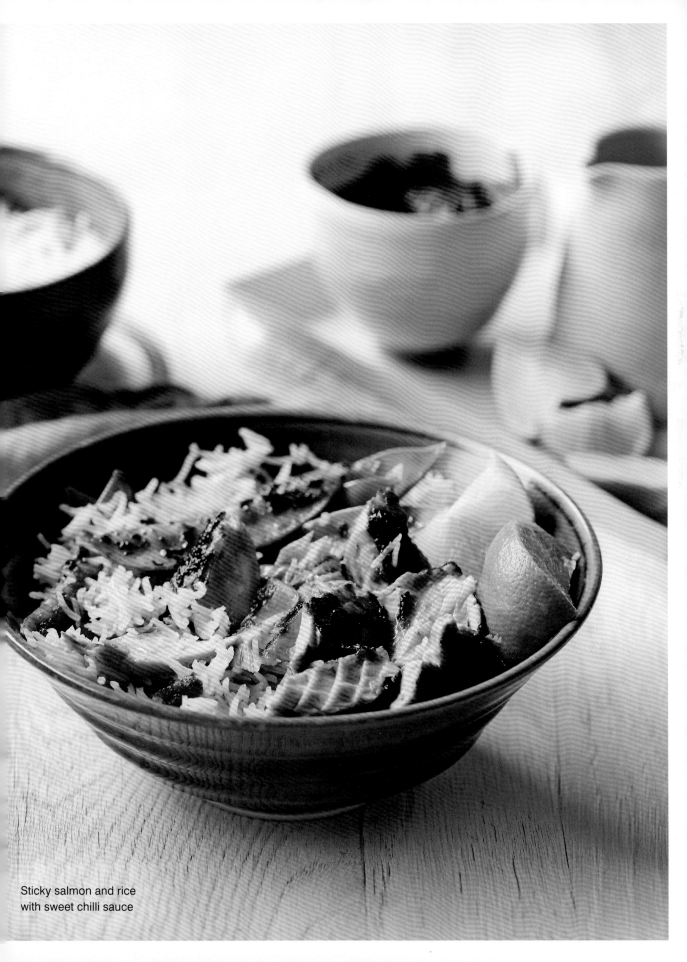

Sticky salmon and rice
with sweet chilli sauce

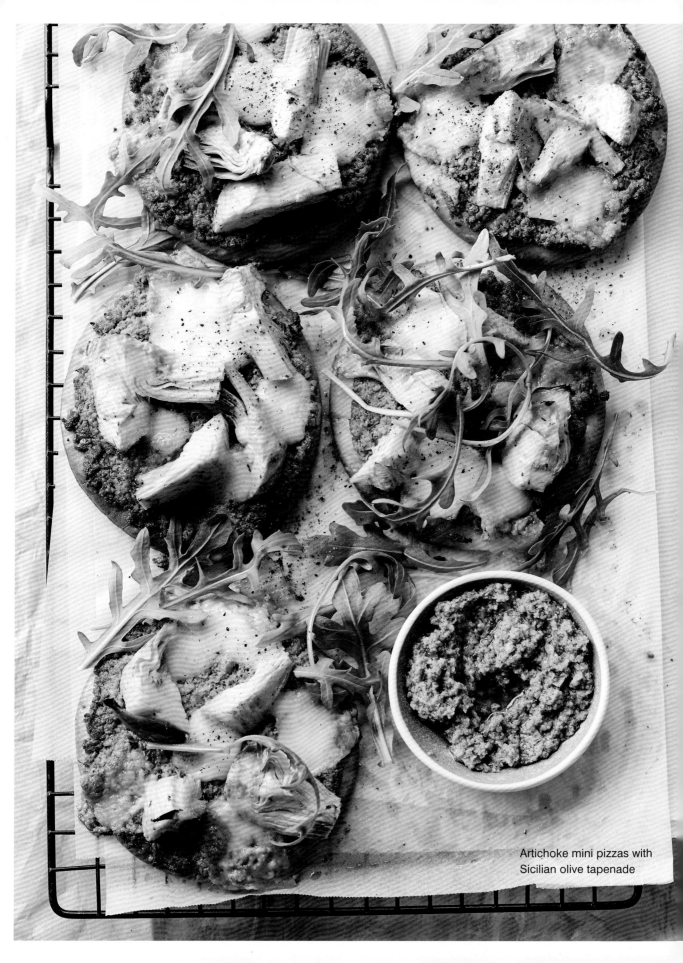

Artichoke mini pizzas with
Sicilian olive tapenade

Sicilian olive tapenade

makes approximately 600 g (1 lb 5 oz/2¼ cups)
preparation 15 minutes

2 small garlic cloves
450 g (1 lb/2 cups) pitted Sicilian green olives
1 tablespoon baby capers, rinsed
zest and juice of 1 lemon
125 ml (4 fl oz/½ cup) extra virgin olive oil

1 Add the garlic, olives and capers to the mixer bowl, measuring cup in. Chop for 10 sec/speed 9. Scrape down the side of the bowl.

2 Add the remaining ingredients to the mixer bowl, measuring cup in. Chop for 20 sec/speed 7.

STORAGE

The tapenade will keep in an airtight container in the fridge for up to 7 days.

TRY THIS

Toss through cooked pasta

Spread over hot toast and top with rocket (arugula) leaves

Spread under the skin of a whole chicken before roasting

Toss through marinara seafood mix before barbecuing

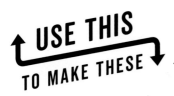

USE THIS TO MAKE THESE

Artichoke mini pizzas

Preheat the oven to 220°C (425°F)/200°C (400°F) fan-forced. Line two large baking trays with baking paper. Place 6 **mini pizza bases** on the prepared trays, then spread evenly with 1 full quantity of the **tapenade**. Top with 500 g (1 lb 2 oz) drained and halved **artichoke hearts**, then 220 g (7¾ oz) torn **bocconcini** (fresh baby mozzarella cheese). Bake for 15 minutes or until until the pizza bases are cooked and crisp and the cheese melts. Serve sprinkled with 50 g (1¾ oz) **baby rocket** (arugula) leaves.

Lamb mini pizzas

Preheat the oven to 220°C (425°F)/200°C (400°F) fan-forced. Line two large baking trays with baking paper. Place 6 **mini pizza bases** on the prepared trays, then spread evenly with 1 full quantity of the **tapenade**. Top with 500 g (1 lb 2 oz) cooked **minced (ground) lamb**, then 200 g (7 oz) crumbled **Danish feta cheese**. Bake for 15 minutes or until the pizza bases are cooked and crisp. Serve sprinkled with 30 g (1 oz/1 cup) **basil leaves**.

Chicken mini pizzas

Preheat the oven to 220°C (425°F)/200°C (400°F) fan-forced. Line two large baking trays with baking paper. Place 6 **mini pizza bases** on the prepared trays, then spread evenly with 1 full quantity of the **tapenade**. Top with 500 g (1 lb 2 oz) shredded **barbecued chicken**, then 120 g (4¼ oz/1 cup) grated **pizza cheese** (mozzarella, cheddar, parmesan). Bake for 15 minutes or until the pizza bases are cooked and crisp and the cheese melts. Serve topped with 200 g (7 oz) sliced **medley baby tomatoes**.

Mustard and mint pickled cucumber

makes approximately 700 g (1 lb 9 oz/2½ cups)
preparation 15 minutes, plus cooling
cooking 10 minutes

2 tablespoons brown mustard seeds
1 teaspoon ground turmeric
80 ml (2½ fl oz/⅓ cup) apple cider vinegar
110 g (3¾ oz/½ cup) white sugar
2 x 250 g (9 oz) baby cucumbers, thinly sliced into rounds
1 small white onion, finely chopped
10 g (¼ oz/¼ cup) small mint leaves

Add the mustard seeds, turmeric, vinegar and sugar to the mixer bowl, measuring cup in. Cook for 10 min/100°C/speed 2 or until the sugar has dissolved. Add the baby cucumbers and onion to the mixer bowl, measuring cup in. Combine for 10 sec/reverse stir/speed 1. Cool the mixture in the mixing bowl. Add the mint to the mixer bowl, measuring cup in. Combine for 10 sec/reverse stir/speed 1.

STORAGE

The pickle will keep in an airtight container in the fridge for up to 7 days (fresh herbs will discolour slightly).

TRY THIS

Use as a dressing for an egg and potato salad

Spoon over poached chicken

Stir through plain Greek-style yoghurt for a dollop sauce

Toss through roasted baby carrots

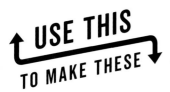

USE THIS TO MAKE THESE

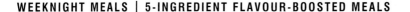

Chicken with carrots

Coat 6 x 120 g (4¼ oz) butterflied skinless **chicken breast fillets** in 2 tablespoons **ground turmeric**. Cook under a grill (broiler) on high for 15 minutes, turning once, until cooked. Combine 1 full quantity of the **pickle** and 2 bunches **baby carrots**, peeled, halved lengthways and blanched. Divide among serving plates, then top with the chicken. Serve dolloped with 130 g (4½ oz/½ cup) **plain Greek-style yoghurt**.

Tofu steaks with radish

Coat 6 x 120 g (4¼ oz) **firm tofu steaks** in 2 tablespoons **ground turmeric**. Cook under a grill (broiler) on high for 10 minutes, turning once, until heated through and golden. Divide 1 full quantity of the **pickle** and 1 bunch **baby radishes**, very thinly sliced, into rounds among serving plates. Top with the **tofu steak**. Serve dolloped with 130 g (4½ oz/½ cup) **plain Greek-style yoghurt**.

Barramundi with beans

Coat 6 x 120 g (4¼ oz) skinless **barramundi fillets** with 2 tablespoons **ground turmeric**. Cook under a grill (broiler) on high for 15 minutes, turning once, until cooked and golden. Divide 1 full quantity of the **pickle** and 500 g (1 lb 2 oz) trimmed and blanched **baby green beans** among serving plates. Top with the barramundi. Serve dolloped with 130 g (4½ oz/½ cup) **plain Greek-style yoghurt**.

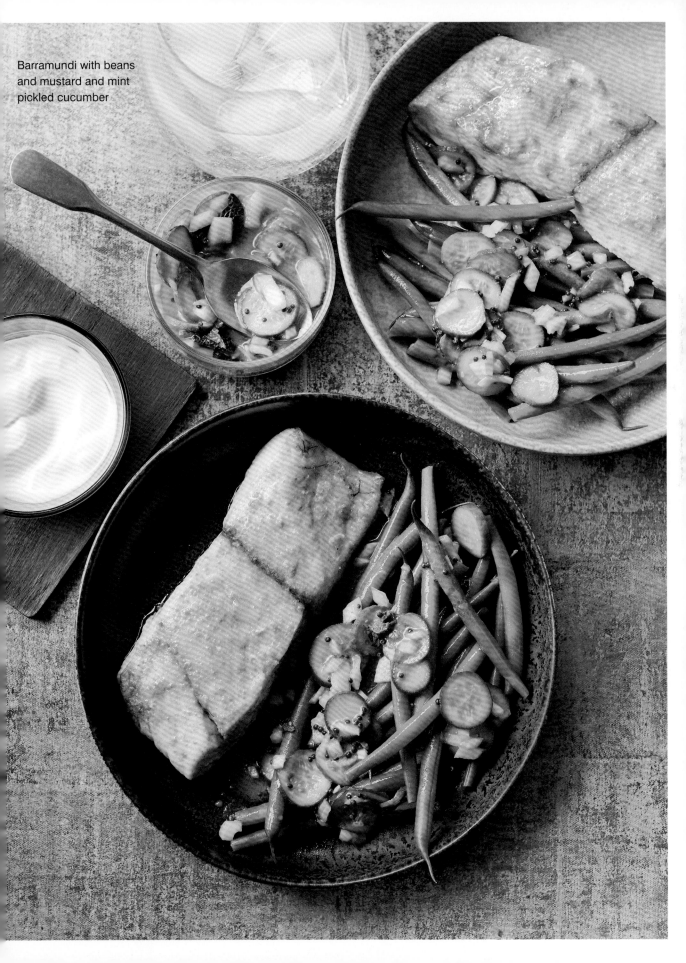

Barramundi with beans
and mustard and mint
pickled cucumber

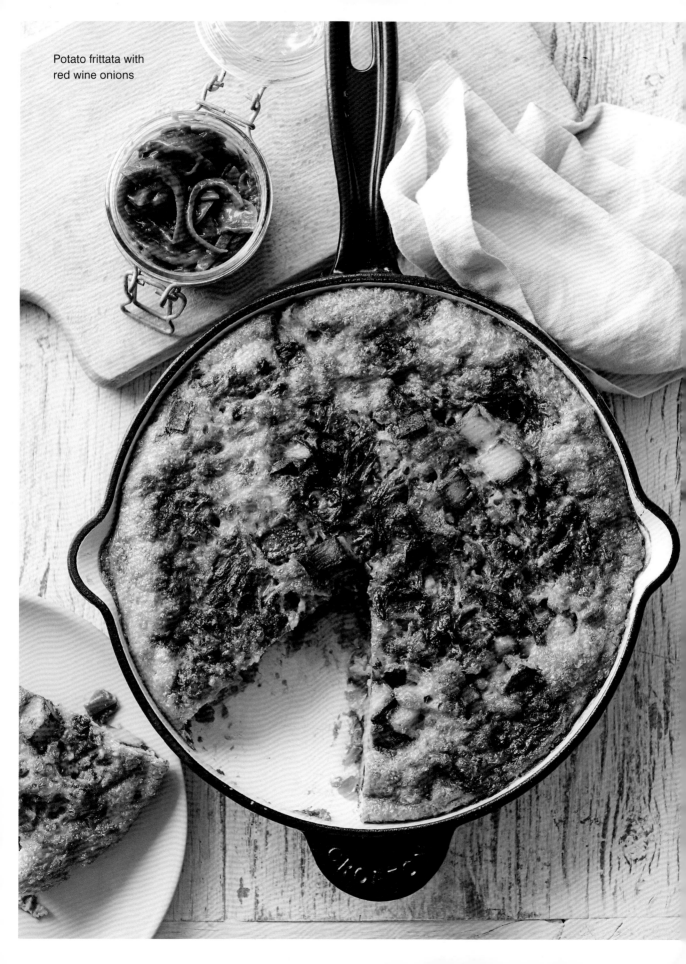

Potato frittata with
red wine onions

Red wine onions

makes approximately 450 g (1 lb/2 cups)
preparation 15 minutes, plus cooling
cooking 35 minutes

50 g (1¾ oz) butter
2 garlic cloves, thinly sliced
3 red onions, thinly sliced
1 tablespoon plain (all-purpose) flour
375 ml (13 fl oz/1½ cups) red wine
1 tablespoon thyme leaves

Place the butter, garlic and onion in the mixer bowl, measuring cup in. Cook for 20 min/100°C/reverse stir/speed 1. Add the remaining ingredients to the mixer bowl, measuring cup removed. Cook for 15 min/steaming temperature/reverse stir/speed 1 or until the mixture is slightly thickened. Use as required or cool completely before storing.

STORAGE

The onions will keep in an airtight container in the fridge for up to 5 days (fresh herbs will discolour slightly).

TRY THIS

Place on sliced bread, top with cheese and grill (broil) to serve alongside soups

Use to layer with minute steaks in a sandwich

Add chicken stock for a simple soup

Dollop over crispy-skin roasted chicken

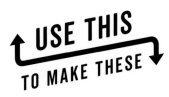

USE THIS TO MAKE THESE

Potato frittata

Heat 80 ml (2½ fl oz/⅓ cup) **olive oil** in a large non-stick frying pan over medium heat. Add 500 g (1 lb 2 oz) peeled and finely chopped all-purpose **potatoes**. Cook, stirring occasionally, for 15 minutes or until golden. Pour over 12 whisked **eggs** combined with 1 full quantity of the **onions**. Reduce the heat to low. Cook, untouched, for 15 minutes or until the frittata is set with a slight wobble in the centre. Place the pan under a grill (broiler) on high to finish cooking the top for 5 minutes or until firm and golden. Stand for 5 minutes before slicing. Serve topped with **basil leaves**.

Chorizo frittata

Heat 80 ml (2½ fl oz/⅓ cup) **olive oil** in a large non-stick frying pan over medium heat. Add 2 finely chopped **cured chorizo**. Cook, stirring occasionally, for 10 minutes or until cooked and golden. Pour over 12 whisked **eggs** combined with 1 full quantity of the **onions**. Reduce the heat to low. Cook, untouched, for 15 minutes or until the frittata is set with a slight wobble in the centre. Place the pan under a grill (broiler) on high to finish cooking the top for 5 minutes or until firm and golden. Stand for 5 minutes before slicing. Serve topped with **baby spinach** (English spinach) leaves.

Chicken frittata

Heat 80 ml (2½ fl oz/⅓ cup) **olive oil** in a non-stick frying pan over medium heat. Add 500 g (1 lb 2 oz) chopped **barbecued chicken**. Cook, stirring occasionally, for 3 minutes or until light golden. Pour over 12 whisked **eggs** combined with 1 full quantity of the **onions**. Reduce the heat to low. Cook, untouched, for 15 minutes or until the frittata is set with a slight wobble in the centre. Sprinkle the top with 200 g (7 oz) crumbled **marinated goat's feta**. Place the pan under a grill (broiler) on high to finish cooking the top for 5 minutes or until firm and golden. Stand for 5 minutes before slicing. Serve.

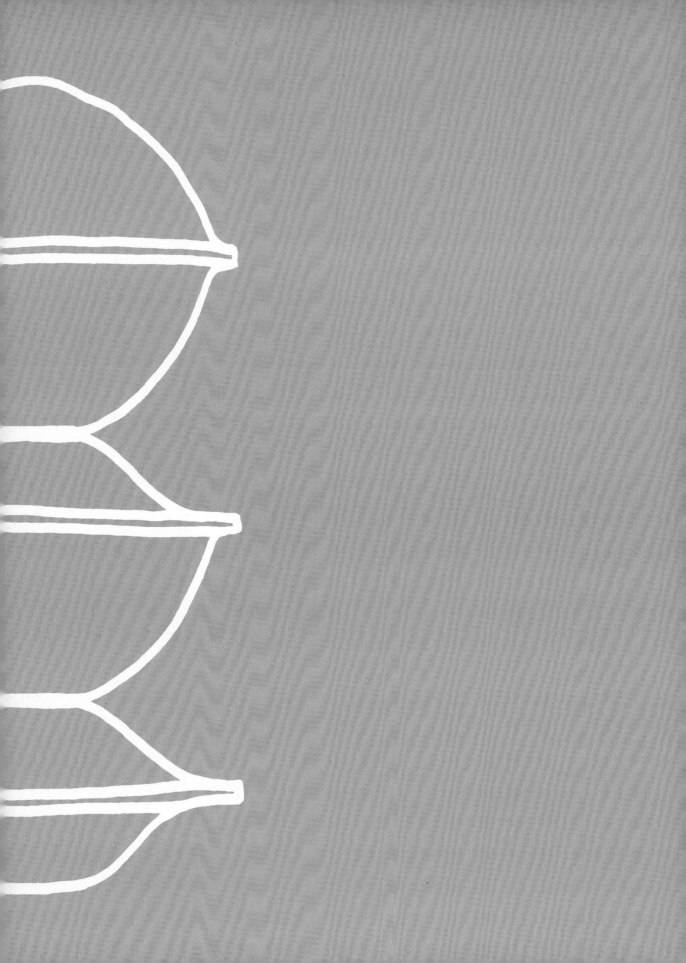

the great batch-cook & freeze chapter

freezer flavour staples

Make midweek meal madness a thing of the past! Roll up your sleeves, don an apron and set aside some cooking time on the weekend to make any of these big-batch freezer meals – either in 12- or 16-serve batches. Spending some time doing this every month or two will ensure your freezer is stocked with portioned-out meals that can be simply reheated and enjoyed in minutes. Don't forget to label and date each container.

In this section you'll see the foundations of the meals are either spice pastes or flavour bases. These are the recipes that we tend to either order from take-out menus or purchase ready-made from the supermarket in jars or sachets. Making these yourself will save you money and give you the reassurance of knowing that you're using fresh ingredients.

The spice paste recipes make enough for 4 x 4-serve meals and the flavour base recipes make enough for 2 x 6-serve meals.

STORING SPICE PASTES

(PAGES 126–29)

1 full quantity
Store in an airtight container in the fridge for up to 1 week.

2 full quantities
Separate into individual serves and store in an airtight container in the freezer for up to 3 months. Defrost in the fridge overnight.

3 to 4 full quantities
Separate into individual serves and store in an airtight container in the freezer for up to 3 months. Defrost in the fridge overnight.

STORING FLAVOUR BASES

(PAGES 130–33)

To store the flavour bases, divide into 6-serve portions, then pop in airtight containers in the fridge for up to 3 days, or freeze for up to 3 months (defrost in the fridge overnight before using). Just remember that once these flavour bases have been stored in the freezer and defrosted to be used, you cannot refreeze them. Make sure to use them within 2 days of defrosting.

STORING 4-SERVE MEALS MADE FROM SPICE PASTES

(PAGES 134–57)

Labelled and dated containers can be stored in the fridge for up to 3 days or in the freezer for up to 3 months. Defrost in the fridge overnight before gently reheating on the stove (adding a little water to loosen if required).

Thai green paste

makes 550 g (1 lb 4 oz/3 cups)
  (4 x 4-serve meals)
preparation 15 minutes

2 garlic cloves
5 cm (2 inch) piece fresh ginger,
  peeled and cut into 4
4 lemongrass stems, white part only,
  cut into 2 cm (¾ inch) lengths
8 fresh kaffir lime leaves, torn
12 spring onions (scallions),
  cut into 4 cm (1½ inch) lengths
8 long fresh green chillies, cut into 4
1 tablespoon Thai spice blend (page 23)
3 small bunches coriander (cilantro),
  washed well, stems and leaves torn
125 ml (4 fl oz/½ cup) macadamia oil

1 Add the garlic, ginger, lemongrass, kaffir lime
   leaves, spring onion, chillies, spice blend and
   coriander to the mixer bowl, measuring cup
   in. Chop for 5 sec/speed 9 and repeat the
   chopping (scraping down the side of the bowl
   each time) until a paste forms.

2 Remove the measuring cup. Mix for 1 min/
   speed 4, while slowly pouring in the oil until
   completely blended.

TRY THIS

Add to white fish before processing
to make fishcakes

**Toss through sliced chicken before
chargrilling**

Cook with coconut cream for a simple
drizzle sauce for roasted meats, chicken
or fish

**Toss through chopped firm tofu
before stir-frying**

Thai red paste

makes 450 g (1 lb/1¾ cups)
  (4 x 4-serve meals)
preparation 15 minutes, plus soaking time

10 dried long red chillies, stems removed
boiling water
2 garlic cloves
2 lemongrass stems, white part only,
  cut into 2 cm (¾ inch) lengths
5 cm (2 inch) piece fresh ginger, peeled
  and cut into 4
2 red onions, quartered
4 fresh long red chillies, cut into 4
1 tablespoon Thai spice blend (page 23)
3 teaspoons dried shrimp paste
80 ml (2½ fl oz/⅓ cup) macadamia oil

1 Soak the dried chillies in a bowl of boiling
   water for 10 minutes to soften. Drain.

2 Add the soaked chillies, garlic, lemongrass,
   ginger, onion, fresh chillies, spice blend and
   shrimp paste to the mixer bowl, measuring cup
   in. Chop for 10 sec/speed 9 and repeat the
   chopping (scraping down the side of the bowl
   each time) until a paste forms.

3 Remove the measuring cup. Mix for 1 min/
   speed 4, while slowly pouring in the oil until
   completely blended.

TRY THIS

Add to foil parcels of vegetables before
baking

**Use to marinate beef steaks before
barbecuing**

Use as a flavour base for laksa

**Mix with crunchy peanut butter,
brown sugar and coconut cream
for an easy satay sauce**

Korma paste

makes 500 g (1 lb 2 oz/2 cups)
  (4 x 4-serve meals)
preparation 15 minutes

4 garlic cloves
7 cm (2¾ inch) piece fresh ginger,
  peeled and cut into 4
1 red onion, quartered
4 long fresh green chillies, cut into 4
50 g (1¾ oz/⅓ cup) raw cashews
45 g (1½ oz/½ cup) desiccated coconut
1 tablespoon Indian spice blend (page 17)
1 tablespoon sweet paprika
125 g (4½ oz/½ cup) tomato paste
  (concentrated purée)
1 small bunch coriander (cilantro), washed
  well, stems and leaves torn
80 ml (2½ fl oz/⅓ cup) macadamia oil

1 Add the garlic, ginger, onion, chillies, cashews,
   coconut, spice blend, paprika, tomato paste and
   coriander to the mixer bowl, measuring cup in.
   Chop for 10 sec/speed 9 and repeat the
   chopping (scraping down the side of the bowl
   each time) until a paste forms.

2 Remove the measuring cup. Mix for 1 min/
   speed 4, while slowly pouring in the oil until
   completely blended.

TRY THIS

Use as a flavour base for split red
lentil dal

**Rub over whole chicken breast fillets
before roasting**

Use as a marinade for threaded firm tofu
and vegie skewers

Add to rice before making a pilaf

Madras paste

makes 430 g (15¼ oz/1¾ cups)
  (4 x 4-serve meals)
preparation 15 minutes

1 tablespoon cumin seeds
1 tablespoon coriander seeds
2 teaspoons black peppercorns
2 tablespoons brown mustard seeds
4 garlic cloves
5 cm (2 inch) piece fresh ginger,
  peeled and cut into 4
1 onion, quartered
1 tablespoon Indian spice blend (page 17)
1 tablespoon ground turmeric
80 ml (2½ fl oz/⅓ cup) malt vinegar
80 ml (2½ fl oz/⅓ cup) macadamia oil

1 Add the cumin seeds, coriander seeds,
   peppercorns and mustard seeds to the mixer
   bowl, measuring cup in. Mill for 1 min/speed 10
   and repeat milling (scraping down the side of the
   bowl each time) until you have a fine powder.

2 Add the garlic, ginger, onion, spice blend
   and turmeric to the mixer bowl, measuring
   cup in. Chop for 10 sec/speed 9 and repeat the
   chopping (scraping down the side of the bowl
   each time) until a paste forms.

3 Add the vinegar to the mixer bowl, measuring
   cup removed. Mix for 1 min/speed 4, while slowly
   pouring in the oil until completely blended.

TRY THIS

Add to cooked minced (ground) beef
for a pie filling

**Add to drained tinned lentils for
a baked potato filler**

Toss through pulled barbecued chicken
for a naan topper

**Use as a flavour base for a hearty
vegetable soup**

Chinese spice paste

makes 500 g (1 lb 2 oz/2 cups)
  (4 x 4-serve meals)
preparation 15 minutes

6 garlic cloves
7 cm (2¾ inch) piece fresh ginger,
  peeled and cut into 4
12 spring onions (scallions),
  cut into 4 cm (1½ inch) lengths
2 tablespoons Chinese spice blend (page 24)
125 ml (4 fl oz/½ cup) soy sauce
2 teaspoons sesame oil
60 ml (2 fl oz/¼ cup) macadamia oil

1 Add the garlic, ginger, spring onion and spice
   blend to the mixer bowl, measuring cup in. Chop
   for 10 sec/speed 9 and repeat the chopping
   (scraping down the side of the bowl each time)
   until a paste forms.

2 Add the soy sauce and sesame oil to the mixer
   bowl, measuring cup removed. Mix for 1 min/
   speed 4, while slowly pouring in the oil until
   completely blended.

TRY THIS

Rub over rolled pork before roasting

**Use to marinate beef strips before
stir-frying**

Mix with vegetable stock to braise Asian
greens

**Mix with plum conserve and use as
a glaze for roasted leg ham**

Italian tomato paste

makes 550 g (1 lb 4 oz/2½ cups)
  (4 x 4-serve meals)
preparation 15 minutes

4 garlic cloves
4 red onions, quartered
420 g (15 oz/2 cups) semi-dried
  (sun-blushed) tomatoes in oil
2 tablespoons Italian spice blend (page 14)
30 g (1 oz/1 cup) basil leaves
zest and juice of 1 lemon
80 ml (2½ fl oz/⅓ cup) extra virgin olive oil

1 Add the garlic, onion, tomatoes, spice blend and
   basil to the mixer bowl, measuring cup in. Chop
   for 10 sec/speed 9 and repeat the chopping
   (scraping down the side of the bowl each time)
   until a paste forms.

2 Add the lemon zest and juice to the mixer bowl,
   measuring cup removed. Mix for 1 min/speed 4,
   while slowly pouring in the oil until completely
   blended.

TRY THIS

Spread over pizza bases before topping
and baking

Toss through any cooked pasta

Use as a flavour base for minestrone

**Spread over toasted ciabatta, then
top with torn bocconcini (fresh baby
mozzarella cheese)**

Harissa paste

makes 350 g (12 oz/1½ cups)
  (4 x 4-serve meals)
preparation 15 minutes

4 garlic cloves
2 red onions, quartered
8 long fresh red chillies, cut into 4
2 tablespoons Moroccan spice blend (page 25)
2 tablespoons tomato paste
  (concentrated purée)
80 ml (2½ fl oz/⅓ cup) extra virgin olive oil

1 Add the garlic, onion, chillies, spice blend and
   tomato paste to the mixer bowl, measuring cup
   in. Chop for 10 sec/speed 9 and repeat the
   chopping (scraping down the side of the bowl
   each time) until a paste forms.

2 Remove the measuring cup. Mix for 1 min/
   speed 4, while slowly pouring in the oil until
   completely blended.

TRY THIS

Rub over mini lamb roasts before baking

Use as a flavour base for vegetable patties

Toss with baby carrots before roasting

Mix with honey and baste salmon fillets before grilling

Smoky paste

makes 625 g (1 lb 6 oz/2½ cups)
  (4 x 4-serve meals)
preparation 15 minutes

4 garlic cloves
2 red onions, quartered
2 long fresh red chillies, cut into 4
445 g (15¾ oz/2 cups) roasted red
  capsicum (pepper)
1 tablespoon dried rosemary
2 tablespoons smoked paprika
80 ml (2½ fl oz/⅓ cup) extra virgin olive oil

1 Add the garlic, onion, chillies, capsicum,
   rosemary and paprika to the mixer bowl,
   measuring cup in. Chop for 10 sec/speed 9
   and repeat the chopping (scraping down the
   side of the bowl each time) until a paste forms.

2 Remove the measuring cup. Mix for 1 min/
   speed 4, while slowly pouring in the oil until
   completely blended.

TRY THIS

Use as a flavour base for homemade baked beans

Toss with pieces of sweet potato before roasting

Use to flavour any meatball mixture

Rub over beef brisket before slow cooking

Honey mustard flavour base

makes 2.25 kg (5 lb/8 cups)
  (2 x 6-serve meals)
preparation 30 minutes
cooking 20 minutes

4 garlic cloves
3 onions, quartered
6 celery stalks, cut into 2 cm (¾ inch) lengths
4 zucchini (courgettes), cut into
  2 cm (¾ inch) lengths
50 g (1¾ oz) butter
60 g (2¼ oz/¼ cup) dijon mustard
80 g (2¾ fl oz/⅓ cup) wholegrain mustard
80 ml (2½ oz/⅓ cup) honey
600 ml (21 fl oz) cream for cooking

1 Add the garlic, onion, celery and zucchini to the mixer bowl, measuring cup in. Chop for 10 sec/speed 7 and repeat the chopping (scraping down the side of the bowl each time) until finely chopped.

2 Add the butter to the mixer bowl, measuring cup in. Cook for 20 min/100°C/speed 1.

3 Add the mustards, honey and cream to the mixer bowl, measuring cup in. Mix for 10 sec/speed 4.

4 Divide the mixture into two equal portions.

TRY THIS Use as a flavour base with pork chipolata sausages, chicken tenderloins, thin beef sausages or firm tofu steaks

Country chicken flavour base

makes approximately 2.4 kg (5 lb 4 oz/8 cups)
  (2 x 6-serve meals)
preparation 30 minutes
cooking 25 minutes

60 ml (2 fl oz/¼ cup) olive oil
2 tablespoons French spice blend (page 21)
4 carrots, chopped into 1 cm (½ inch) dice
2 leeks, white part only, thinly sliced
4 celery stalks, cut into 1 cm (½ inch) dice
500 g (1 lb 2 oz) peeled pumpkin (squash),
  cut into 1 cm (½ inch) dice
1 tablespoon thyme leaves
375 ml (13 fl oz/1½ cups) white wine
300 ml (10½ fl oz) cream for cooking
500 g (1 lb 2 oz/2⅓ cups) frozen baby peas

1 Add the oil, spice blend, carrot, leek, celery, pumpkin and thyme to the mixer bowl, measuring cup in. Cook for 15 min/100°C/reverse stir/speed 1.

2 Add the wine to the mixer bowl, measuring cup removed. Cook for 10 min/100°C/reverse stir/speed 2.

3 Add the cream to the mixer bowl, measuring cup removed. Mix for 10 sec/reverse stir/speed 4.

4 Transfer the mixture to a large heatproof bowl. Add the peas. Mix well to combine.

5 Divide the mixture into two equal portions.

TRY THIS Use as a flavour base with chicken breast, chicken thigh, chicken tenderloins or pork fillet

Farmhouse ragu flavour base

makes approximately 2.4 kg (5 lb 4 oz/8 cups)
  (2 x 6-serve meals)
preparation 30 minutes
cooking 25 minutes

4 garlic cloves
3 red onions, quartered
4 carrots, cut into 2 cm (¾ inch) lengths
4 zucchini (courgettes), cut into 2 cm (¾ inch)
  lengths
60 ml (2 fl oz/¼ cup) olive oil
2 tablespoons Italian spice blend (page 14)
90 g (3 oz/⅓ cup) tomato paste
  (concentrated purée)
500 ml (17 fl oz/2 cups) red wine
800 g (1 lb 12 oz) tinned chopped tomatoes
250 ml (9 fl oz/1 cup) vegetable stock
2 tablespoons chopped rosemary leaves

1 Add the garlic, onion, carrot and zucchini to
   the mixer bowl, measuring cup in. Chop for
   10 sec/speed 7 and repeat the chopping
   (scraping down the side of the bowl each
   time) until finely chopped.

2 Add the oil, spice blend and tomato paste
   to the mixer bowl, measuring cup in. Cook for
   3 min/100°C/speed 2.

3 Add the wine to the mixer bowl, measuring cup
   in. Cook for 10 min/100°C/speed 2.

4 Add the tomatoes, stock and rosemary to
   the mixer bowl, measuring cup in and the
   steamer basket set over the lid. Cook for
   10 min/100°C/speed 2.

5 Divide the mixture into two equal portions.

TRY THIS Use as a flavour base with beef blade
steak, lamb shoulder, chicken thigh
or beef chuck steak

Chinese chow mein flavour base

makes 1.8 kg (4 lb/6 cups)
  (2 x 6-serve meals)
preparation 30 minutes
cooking 20 minutes

4 garlic cloves
60 ml (2 fl oz/¼ cup) macadamia oil
3 onions, cut into thin wedges
80 ml (2½ fl oz/⅓ cup) soy sauce
125 ml (4 fl oz/½ cup) oyster sauce
250 ml (9 fl oz/1 cup) vegetable stock
4 zucchini (courgettes), chopped
3 red capsicums (peppers), chopped
8 spring onions (scallions), thinly sliced

1 Add the garlic to the mixer bowl, measuring cup
   in. Chop for 10 sec/speed 7. Scrape down the
   side of the bowl.

2 Add the oil and onion to the mixer bowl,
   measuring cup in. Cook for 3 min/100°C/
   reverse stir/speed 2.

3 Add the sauces, stock, zucchini and capsicum
   to the mixer bowl, measuring cup removed
   and the steamer basket set over the lid. Cook
   for 15 min/100°C/reverse stir/speed 1.

4 Add the spring onion to the mixer bowl,
   measuring cup in. Mix for 10 sec/reverse stir/
   speed 4.

5 Divide the mixture into two equal portions.

TRY THIS Use as a flavour base with
vegetarian/vegan 'mince', beef
strips, lamb backstrap (loin fillet)
or minced (ground) chicken

Sweet and sour flavour base

makes 2.5 kg (5 lb 8 oz/10 cups)
  (2 x 6-serve meals)
preparation 30 minutes
cooking 20 minutes

3 garlic cloves
5 cm (2 inch) piece fresh ginger,
  peeled and halved
60 ml (2 fl oz/¼ cup) macadamia oil
3 red onions, chopped
4 green capsicums (peppers), chopped
3 carrots, halved lengthways and
  sliced diagonally
2 tablespoons cornflour (cornstarch)
850 g (1 lb 14 oz) tinned pineapple pieces
  in natural juice
80 ml (2½ fl oz/⅓ cup) soy sauce
80 ml (2½ fl oz/⅓ cup) white vinegar
80 ml (2½ fl oz/⅓ cup) tomato sauce (ketchup)

1 Add the garlic and ginger to the mixer bowl,
   measuring cup in. Chop for 10 sec/speed 7.
   Scrape down the side of the bowl.

2 Add the oil and onion to the mixer bowl,
   measuring cup in. Cook for 3 min/100°C/
   reverse stir/speed 2.

3 Add the remaining ingredients to the mixer
   bowl, measuring cup in. Cook for 15 min/100°C/
   reverse stir/speed 1.

4 Divide the mixture into two equal portions.

TRY THIS Use as a flavour base with pork
fillet, firm white fish fillets, firm tofu
or chicken breast

Hotpot flavour base

makes 2.25 kg (5 lb/8 cups)
  (2 x 6-serve meals)
preparation 30 minutes
cooking 20 minutes

4 garlic cloves
2 tablespoons rosemary leaves
3 onions, quartered
4 carrots, cut into 2 cm (¾ inch) pieces
60 ml (2 fl oz/¼ cup) extra virgin olive oil
2 tablespoons All-purpose spice blend (page 22)
250 ml (9 fl oz/1 cup) vegetable stock
400 g (14 oz) green beans, cut into 2 cm
  (¾ inch) lengths
410 g (14½ oz) tinned apricot halves in juice
2 tablespoons honey

1 Add the garlic, rosemary, onion and carrot to the
   mixer bowl, measuring cup in. Chop for 10 sec/
   speed 7. Repeat the chopping (scraping down
   the side of the bowl) until finely chopped.

2 Add the oil and spice blend to the mixer bowl,
   measuring cup in. Cook for 15 min/100°C/speed 2.
   Scrape down the side of the bowl.

3 Add the stock and beans to the mixer bowl,
   measuring cup in. Cook for 5 min/100°C/
   reverse stir/speed 1. Scrape down the side of
   the bowl.

4 Add the apricots and their juice and the honey to
   the mixer bowl, measuring cup in. Mix for 10 sec/
   reverse stir/speed 2. Scrape down the side of
   the bowl.

5 Divide the mixture into two equal portions.

TRY THIS Use as a flavour base with lamb
backstrap (loin fillet), beef topside,
chicken breast or beef or chicken
sausages

Chicken cacciatore flavour base

makes 2.25 kg (5 lb/8 cups)
  (2 x 6-serve meals)
preparation 30 minutes
cooking 30 minutes

3 garlic cloves
3 red onions, quartered
60 ml (2 fl oz/¼ cup) extra virgin olive oil
6 anchovy fillets
90 g (3 oz/⅓ cup) tomato paste
  (concentrated purée)
250 ml (9 fl oz/1 cup) white wine
800 g (1 lb 12 oz) tinned chopped tomatoes
150 g (5½ oz) diced pancetta
600 g (1 lb 5 oz) small button mushrooms
180 g (6½ oz/⅔ cup) pitted kalamata olives
15 g (½ oz/½ cup) chopped flat-leaf (Italian) parsley
7 g (¼ oz/¼ cup) oregano leaves

1 Add the garlic and onion to the mixer bowl, measuring cup in. Chop for 10 sec/speed 7 and repeat the chopping (scraping down the side of the bowl each time) until finely chopped.

2 Add the oil, anchovies and tomato paste to the mixer bowl, measuring cup in. Cook for 3 min/100°C/speed 2. Add the wine, measuring cup removed. Cook for 10 min/100°C/speed 2.

3 Add the tomatoes, pancetta, mushrooms and olives to the mixer bowl, measuring cup removed and the steamer basket placed on the lid. Cook for 15 min/100°C/reverse stir/speed 1. Add the parsley and oregano to the mixer bowl, measuring cup in. Mix for 10 sec/reverse stir/speed 4. Divide the mixture into two equal portions.

TRY THIS Use as a flavour base with chicken or pork

Mild coconut curry flavour base

makes 2.25 kg (5 lb/8 cups)
  (2 x 6-serve meals)
preparation 30 minutes
cooking 20 minutes

3 garlic cloves
6 spring onions (scallions), cut into
  4 cm lengths
6 celery stalks, cut into 2 cm (¾ inch) lengths
6 carrots, cut into 2 cm (¾ inch) lengths
4 zucchini (courgettes), cut into 2 cm
  (¾ inch) lengths
60 ml (2 fl oz/¼ cup) macadamia oil
1 tablespoon Indian spice blend (page 17)
800 ml (28 fl oz) tinned coconut cream
15 g (½ oz/½ cup) coriander (cilantro) leaves

1 Add the garlic, spring onion, celery, carrot and zucchini to the mixer bowl, measuring cup in. Chop for 10 sec/speed 7 and repeat the chopping (scraping down the side of the bowl each time) until finely chopped.

2 Add the oil and spice blend to the mixer bowl, measuring cup in. Cook for 2 min/100°C/speed 1.

3 Add the coconut cream to the mixer bowl, measuring cup in. Cook for 15 min/100°C/speed 1.

4 Add the coriander to the mixer bowl, measuring cup in. Mix for 10 sec/speed 4.

5 Divide the mixture into two equal portions.

TRY THIS Use as a flavour base with chicken breast, firm white fish fillets, raw peeled prawns (shrimp) or beef or chicken sausages

Thai chicken green curry

serves 16 (4 x 4-serve meals)
preparation 45 minutes, plus 15 minutes standing time
cooking 50 minutes

125 ml (4 fl oz/½ cup) macadamia oil
2.5 kg (5 lb 8 oz) chicken stir-fry strips
1 full quantity Thai green paste (page 126)
1.6 litres (55½ fl oz) tinned coconut milk
45 g (1½ oz/¼ cup) brown sugar
2 tablespoons fish sauce
juice of 4 limes
8 zucchini (courgettes), halved lengthways,
  then thickly sliced
800 g (1 lb 12 oz) sugar snap peas, trimmed
15 g (½ oz/½ cup) coriander (cilantro) leaves
  (optional)
rice, noodles or steamed Asian greens, to serve

1 Preheat a large stockpot over high heat. Place the oil and chicken
   in a large bowl, tossing well to combine and coat evenly.

2 Cook the chicken in the pot, in eight batches, for 5 minutes each, until
   almost cooked and light golden. Transfer each batch of chicken to a
   large heatproof bowl and reheat the stockpot until hot before browning
   the next batch.

3 Meanwhile, add the green paste, coconut milk, sugar, fish sauce
   and lime juice to the mixer bowl, measuring cup in. Cook for 10 min/
   100°C/speed 1.

4 Return all the chicken, and any resting juices, to the pot. Add the paste
   mixture. Stir until the mixture just comes to the boil, then reduce the
   heat to medium. Add the zucchini. Cook, stirring occasionally, for
   10 minutes or until the chicken is cooked and the zucchini is just tender.

5 Remove the pot from the heat. Add the sugar snaps and coriander
   and stir to combine. Stand, covered, for 15 minutes. Divide the mixture
   evenly among four airtight containers to store.

6 Serve with rice, your favourite noodles or simple steamed
   Asian greens.

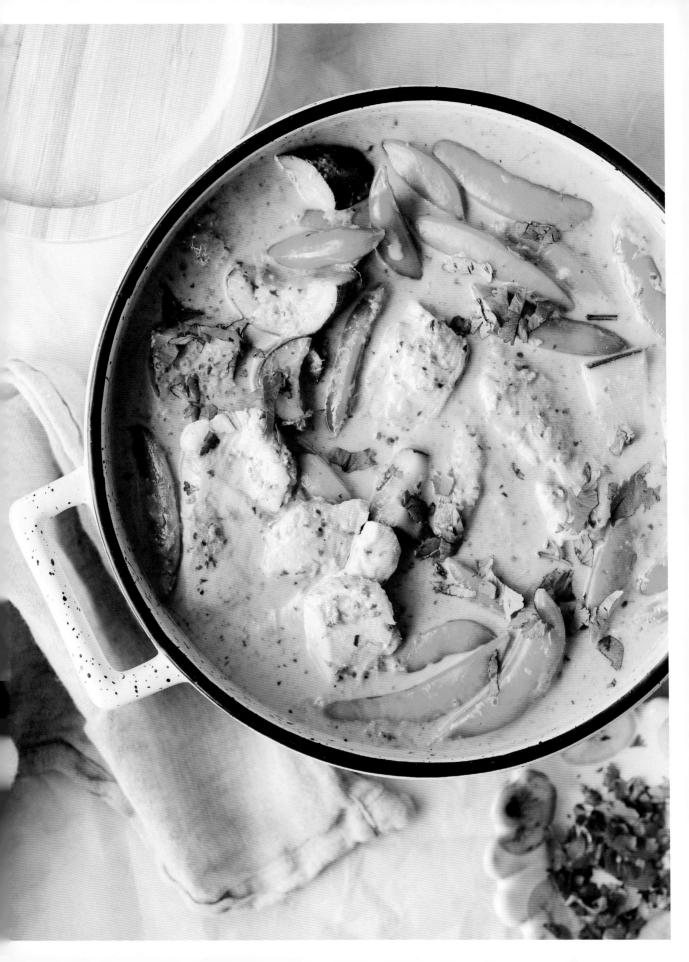

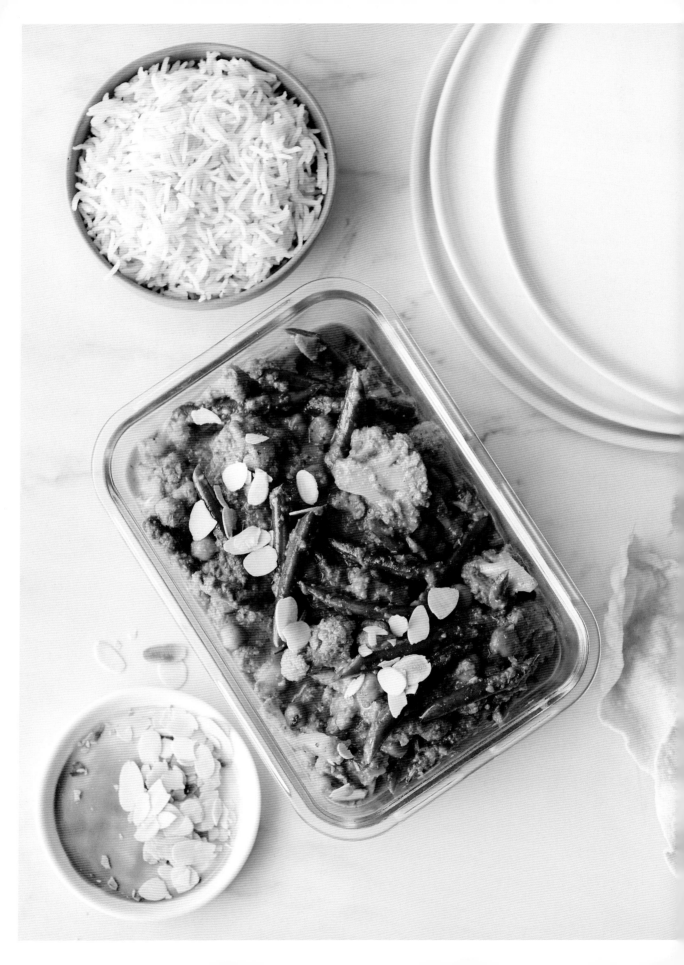

Chickpea and vegetable korma

serves 16 (4 x 4-serve meals)
preparation 45 minutes, plus 15 minutes standing time
cooking 30 minutes

4 red onions, quartered
125 ml (4 fl oz/½ cup) macadamia oil
1 full quantity Korma paste (page 127)
500 ml (17 fl oz/2 cups) vegetable stock
600 ml (21 fl oz) cream for cooking
1.6 kg (3 lb 8 oz) tinned chickpeas, drained and rinsed
1.5 kg (3 lb 5 oz) cauliflower florets, broken into 3 cm
  (1¼ inch) pieces
800 g (1 lb 12 oz) green beans, trimmed and halved
50 g (1¾ oz/½ cup) toasted almond flakes (optional)
rice, naan or poppadoms, to serve

1 Add the onion to the mixer bowl, measuring cup in. Chop for 5 sec/
   speed 7. Scrape down the side of the bowl. Chop for 3 sec/speed 5.
   Scrape down the side of the bowl.

2 Add the oil to the mixer bowl, measuring cup in. Cook for 10 min/100°C/
   speed 1.

3 Add the korma paste, stock and cream to the mixer bowl, measuring
   cup in. Heat for 2 min/100°C/speed 1.

4 Pour the mixture into a large stockpot and place over medium heat.
   Bring to a simmer.

5 Add the chickpeas and cauliflower to the pot. Cook, stirring
   occasionally, for 15 minutes or until the cauliflower is just tender.

6 Remove the pot from the heat. Add the beans and almonds (if using)
   and stir to combine. Stand, covered, for 15 minutes. Divide the mixture
   evenly among four airtight containers to store.

7 Serve with rice, naan or poppadoms.

Beef madras

serves 16 (4 x 4-serve meals)
preparation 50 minutes, plus 15 minutes standing time
cooking 2 hours 40 minutes

4 onions, quartered
6 garlic cloves
5 cm (2 inch) piece fresh ginger, peeled and halved
125 ml (4 fl oz/½ cup) macadamia oil
2.5 kg (5 lb 8 oz) lean gravy beef, trimmed and
   cut into 3 cm (1¼ inch) pieces
1 full quantity Madras paste (page 127)
12 cardamom pods, bruised
1 litre (35 fl oz/4 cups) beef stock
1.6 kg (3 lb 8 oz) tinned chopped tomatoes
1.5 kg (3 lb 5 oz) peeled, seeded pumpkin (squash),
   cut into 3 cm (1¼ inch) pieces
300 g (10½ oz) baby spinach (English spinach) leaves
rice, naan or poppadoms, to serve

1   Add the onion, garlic and ginger to the mixer bowl, measuring cup in.
    Chop for 5 sec/speed 7. Scrape down the side of the bowl. No need
    to clean the bowl.

2   Preheat a large stockpot over high heat. Place the onion mixture, oil
    and beef in a large bowl, tossing well to combine and coat evenly.

3   Cook the beef in the stockpot, in eight batches, for 5 minutes each
    until almost cooked and light golden. Transfer each batch of beef to
    a large heatproof bowl and reheat the pot until hot before browning
    the next batch.

4   Meanwhile, add the Madras paste, cardamom pods and stock to the
    mixer bowl, measuring cup in. Cook for 10 min/100°C/speed 1.

5   Return all the beef, and any resting juices, to the pot. Add the paste
    mixture. Stir until the mixture just comes to the boil, then reduce the
    heat to medium–low. Cook, covered and stirring occasionally, for
    1 hour. Add the tomatoes and pumpkin. Cook, covered and stirring
    occasionally, for 1 hour or until the beef is very tender and the
    sauce reduced.

6   Remove the pot from the heat. Add the spinach and stir to combine.
    Stand, covered, for 15 minutes. Divide the mixture evenly among four
    airtight containers to store. Serve with rice, naan or poppadoms.

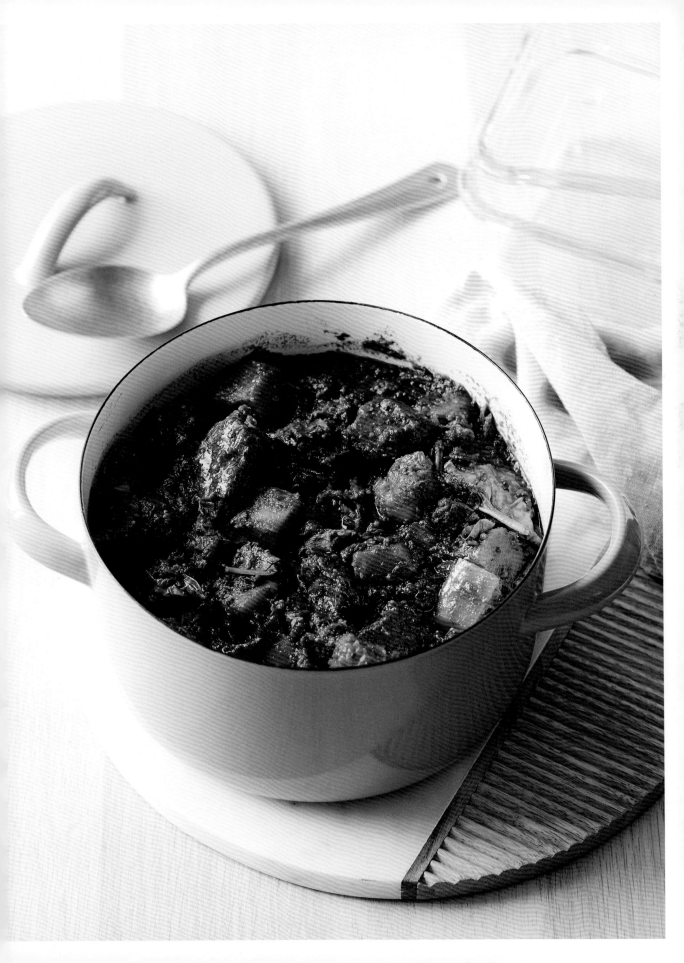

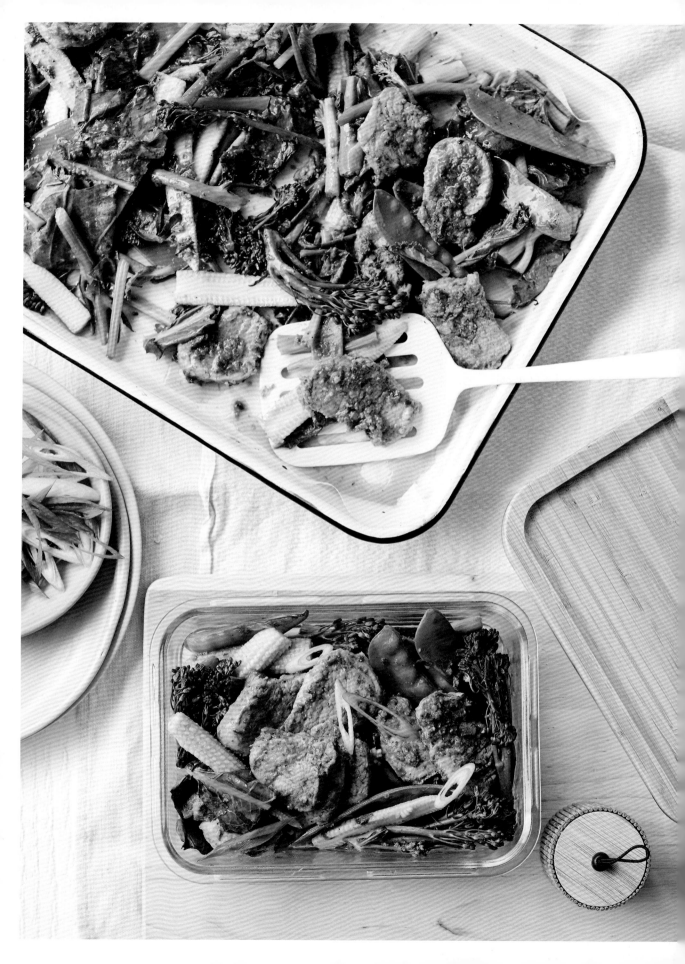

Chinese spice pork

serves 16 (4 x 4-serve meals)
preparation 45 minutes, plus 15 minutes standing time
cooking 35 minutes

4 red onions, thinly sliced
125 ml (4 fl oz/½ cup) macadamia oil
2.5 kg (5 lb 8 oz) pork fillet, trimmed and thinly sliced
1 full quantity Chinese spice paste (page 128)
250 ml (9 fl oz/1 cup) chicken stock
4 bunches broccolini, trimmed and halved crossways
2 bunches Chinese broccoli (gai larn), trimmed,
  then cut into 4 cm (1½ inch) lengths
500 g (1 lb 2 oz) baby corn, halved lengthways
1 kg (2 lb 4 oz) snow peas (mangetout), trimmed
rice, thin egg noodles or hokkien (egg) noodles, to serve

1   Preheat the oven to 200°C (400°F)/180°C (350°F) fan-forced.

2   Add the onion to the mixer bowl, measuring cup in. Chop for 5 sec/
    speed 7. Scrape down the side of the bowl. Chop for 3 sec/speed 5.
    Scrape down the side of the bowl. No need to clean the bowl.

3   Preheat a large wok over high heat. Place the onion mixture, oil and
    pork in a large bowl, tossing well to combine and coat evenly.

4   Stir-fry the pork, in 10 batches, for 2 minutes each until almost cooked
    and light golden. Transfer each batch of pork to a large heatproof bowl
    and reheat the wok until hot before browning the next batch.

5   Meanwhile, add the spice paste and stock to the mixer bowl, measuring
    cup in. Cook for 10 min/100°C/speed 1.

6   Divide the broccolini, Chinese broccoli, baby corn, snow peas and pork
    evenly among two large, deep roasting tins lined with baking paper.
    Evenly pour over the paste mixture. Cover the tins with a piece of
    baking paper, then doubled sheets of foil.

7   Bake in the oven for 15 minutes. Remove from the oven. Stand,
    covered, for 15 minutes. Divide the mixture evenly among four airtight
    containers to store.

8   Serve with rice, thin egg noodles or hokkien (egg) noodles.

Thai beef red curry

serves 16 (4 x 4-serve meals)
preparation 45 minutes, plus 15 minutes standing time
cooking 50 minutes

125 ml (4 fl oz/½ cup)
  macadamia oil
2.5 kg (5 lb 8 oz) beef stir-fry
  strips
1 full quantity Thai red paste
  (page 126)
1.6 litres (55½ fl oz) tinned
  coconut cream
45 g (1½ oz/¼ cup)
  brown sugar
2 tablespoons fish sauce

juice of 4 limes
1.5 kg (3 lb 5 oz) peeled,
  seeded pumpkin (squash),
  cut into 1 cm (½ inch)
  pieces
2 large red capsicums
  (peppers), sliced
75 g (2½ oz/½ cup) chopped
  roasted peanuts (optional)
rice, noodles or steamed
  Asian greens, to serve

1 Preheat a large stockpot over high heat. Place the oil and beef in
   a large bowl, tossing well to combine and coat evenly.

2 Cook the beef in the pot, in eight batches, for 5 minutes each until
   almost cooked and light golden. Transfer each batch of beef to a
   large heatproof bowl and reheat the pot until hot before browning the
   next batch.

3 Meanwhile, add the red paste, coconut cream, sugar, fish sauce and
   lime juice to the mixer bowl, measuring cup in. Cook for 10 min/100°C/
   speed 1.

4 Return all the beef, and any resting juices, to the pot. Add the paste
   mixture. Stir until the mixture just comes to the boil, then reduce the
   heat to medium. Add the pumpkin. Cook, stirring occasionally, for
   10 minutes or until the beef is cooked and the pumpkin is just tender.

5 Remove the pot from the heat. Add the capsicum and peanuts (if using)
   and stir to combine. Stand, covered, for 15 minutes. Divide the mixture
   evenly among four airtight containers to store.

6 Serve with rice, your favourite noodles or steamed Asian greens.

Harissa chicken

serves 16 (4 x 4-serve meals)
preparation 45 minutes, plus 15 minutes standing time
cooking 2 hours 15 minutes

4 red onions, cut into
  thin wedges
8 zucchini (courgettes),
  sliced into rounds
8 carrots, sliced into rounds
125 ml (4 fl oz/½ cup) olive oil
2.5 kg (5 lb 8 oz) skinless
  chicken thigh fillets,
  trimmed and cut into 3
1 full quantity Harissa paste
  (page 129)

2 litres (70 fl oz/8 cups)
  chicken stock
800 g (1 lb 12 oz) tinned
  chopped tomatoes
250 g (9 oz) soft and juicy
  dried figs, halved
juice and finely grated zest
  of 2 lemons
rice, couscous or mashed
  potato, to serve

1 Add the onion to the mixer bowl, measuring cup in. Chop for 5 sec/
   speed 7. Scrape down the side of the bowl. Chop for 3 sec/speed 5, or
   until finely chopped. Transfer to a stockpot. No need to clean the bowl.

2 Add half the zucchini to the mixer bowl, measuring cup in. Chop for
   5 sec/speed 7. Scrape down the side of the bowl. Chop for 3 sec/
   speed 5, or until finely chopped. Transfer to the pot, then chop the
   remaining zucchini. Chop for 5 sec/speed 7. Scrape down the side
   of the bowl. Chop for 3 sec/speed 5, or until finely chopped. Transfer
   to the pot. No need to clean the bowl.

3 Add half the carrot to the mixer bowl, measuring cup in. Chop for 5 sec/
   speed 7. Scrape down the side of the bowl. Chop for 3 sec/speed 5,
   or until finely chopped. Transfer to the pot, then chop the remaining
   carrot. Chop for 5 sec/speed 7. Scrape down the side of the bowl. Chop
   for 3 sec/speed 5, or until finely chopped. Transfer to the pot. Add the
   oil to the pot and place over high heat. Cook, stirring occasionally, for
   15 minutes or until softened. Add the chicken and cook, stirring
   occasionally, for 20 minutes or until light golden.

4 Add the harissa paste, stock and tomatoes to the pot. Reduce the
   heat to medium. Simmer, partially covered and stirring occasionally,
   for 1 hour. Add the figs. Cook, stirring occasionally, for 30 minutes or
   until the chicken is falling apart and the sauce reduces and thickens.
   Remove the pot from the heat. Add the lemon juice and zest and stir to
   combine. Stand, uncovered, for 15 minutes. Divide the mixture evenly
   among four airtight containers to store. Serve with rice, couscous or
   mashed potato.

Italian beef

serves 16 (4 x 4-serve meals)
preparation 30 minutes, plus 15 minutes standing time
cooking 1 hour 45 minutes

4 onions, quartered
6 celery stalks, cut into 2 cm
  (¾ inch) pieces
8 carrots, cut into 2 cm (¾ inch)
  pieces
125 ml (4 fl oz/½ cup) olive oil
2.5 kg (5 lb 8 oz) lean minced
  (ground) beef
1 full quantity Italian tomato
  paste (page 128)

1 litre (35 fl oz/4 cups) beef
  stock
1.6 kg (3 lb 8 oz) tinned
  chopped tomatoes
20 g (¾ oz/1 cup) flat-leaf
  (Italian) parsley leaves
  (optional)
pasta (shapes, filled
  or lasagne), rice or
  mashed potato, to serve

1 Add the onion to the mixer bowl, measuring cup in. Chop for 5 sec/
   speed 7. Scrape down the side of the bowl. Chop for 3 sec/speed 5,
   or until finely chopped. Transfer to a large stockpot. No need to clean
   the bowl.

2 Add the celery to the mixer bowl, measuring cup in. Chop for 5 sec/
   speed 7. Scrape down the side of the bowl. Chop for 3 sec/speed 5,
   or until finely chopped. Transfer to the pot. No need to clean the bowl.

3 Add half the carrot to the mixer bowl, measuring cup in. Chop for 5 sec/
   speed 7. Scrape down the side of the bowl. Chop for 3 sec/speed 5,
   or until finely chopped. Transfer to the pot, then chop the remaining
   carrot. Chop for 5 sec/speed 7. Scrape down the side of the bowl.
   Chop for 3 sec/speed 5, or until finely chopped. Transfer to the pot.

4 Add the oil to the pot and place over high heat. Cook, stirring
   occasionally, for 15 minutes or until softened. Add the beef, cook,
   stirring occasionally and breaking up any lumps with a spoon, for
   30 minutes or until cooked and golden.

5 Add the tomato paste, stock and tomatoes to the pot. Reduce the
   heat to medium. Simmer, partially covered and stirring occasionally,
   for 1 hour or until the sauce reduces and thickens.

6 Remove the pot from the heat. Add the parsley (if using) and stir to
   combine. Stand, uncovered, for 15 minutes. Divide the mixture evenly
   among four airtight containers to store.

7 Serve with pasta, rice or mashed potato.

Spanish sausages

serves 16 (4 x 4-serve meals)
preparation 45 minutes, plus 15 minutes standing time
cooking 55 minutes

4 red onions, quartered
6 celery stalks, cut into 2 cm
  (¾ inch) pieces
8 carrots, cut into 2 cm (¾ inch)
  pieces
125 ml (4 fl oz/½ cup) olive oil
2 kg (4 lb 8 oz) beef chipolatas
1 full quantity Smoky paste
  (page 129)

500 ml (17 fl oz/2 cups) beef
  stock
1.6 kg (14 oz) tinned chopped
  tomatoes
1 kg (2 lb 4 oz) frozen baby peas
rice, couscous or mashed
  potato, to serve

1   Preheat the oven to 200°C (400°F)/180°C (350°F) fan-forced.

2   Add the onion to the mixer bowl, measuring cup in. Chop for 5 sec/
    speed 7. Scrape down the side of the bowl. Chop for 3 sec/speed 5, or until
    finely chopped. Transfer to a large stockpot. No need to clean the bowl.

3   Add the celery to the mixer bowl, measuring cup in. Chop for 5 sec/
    speed 7. Scrape down the side of the bowl. Chop for 3 sec/speed 5,
    or until finely chopped. Transfer to the pot. No need to clean the bowl.

4   Add half the carrot to the mixer bowl, measuring cup in. Chop for
    5 sec/speed 7. Scrape down the side of the bowl. Chop for 3 sec/speed
    5, or until finely chopped. Transfer to the pot, then chop the remaining
    carrot. Chop for 5 sec/speed 7. Scrape down the side of the bowl.
    Chop for 3 sec/speed 5, or until finely chopped. Transfer to the pot.

5   Add the oil to the pot and place over high heat. Cook, stirring
    occasionally, for 15 minutes or until softened.

6   Meanwhile, heat a large non-stick frying pan over medium–high heat
    and brown the chipolatas, in four batches, for 3 minutes each. Transfer
    to a plate.

7   Add the smoky paste and stock to the mixer bowl, measuring cup in.
    Cook for 10 min/100°C/speed 1.

8   Divide the vegetable mixture, the browned chipolatas, the paste mixture
    and the tomatoes evenly between two large roasting tins. Cover the tins
    with a piece of baking paper, then doubled sheets of foil. Bake in the
    oven for 30 minutes. Remove from the oven and add the peas. Stand,
    covered, for 15 minutes. Divide the mixture evenly among four airtight
    containers to store. Serve with rice, couscous or mashed potato.

Country chicken

serves 12 (3 x 4-serve meals)
preparation 40 minutes, plus 15 minutes standing time
cooking 50 minutes

80 ml (2½ fl oz/⅓ cup) olive oil
1.8 kg (4 lb) skinless chicken breast fillets,
  cut into 2 cm (¾ inch) pieces
500 ml (17 fl oz/2 cups) chicken stock
1 full quantity Country chicken flavour base (page 130)
10 g (¼ oz/½ cup) chopped flat-leaf (Italian) parsley
pasta shapes, rice or mashed potato, to serve

1 Preheat a large heavy-based saucepan over high heat. Place the oil
   and chicken in a large bowl, tossing well to combine and coat evenly.

2 Cook the chicken in the pan, in six batches, for 5 minutes each until
   almost cooked and light golden. Transfer each batch of chicken to a
   large heatproof bowl and reheat the pan until hot before browning the
   next batch.

3 Return all the chicken, and any resting juices, to the pan. Add the stock
   and flavour base. Stir until the mixture just comes to the boil, then
   reduce the heat to medium. Cook, stirring occasionally, for 20 minutes
   or until the chicken is cooked and the sauce has thickened slightly.

4 Remove the pan from the heat. Add the parsley and stir to combine.
   Stand, covered, for 15 minutes. Divide the mixture evenly among four
   airtight containers to store.

5 Serve with pasta shapes, rice or mashed potato.

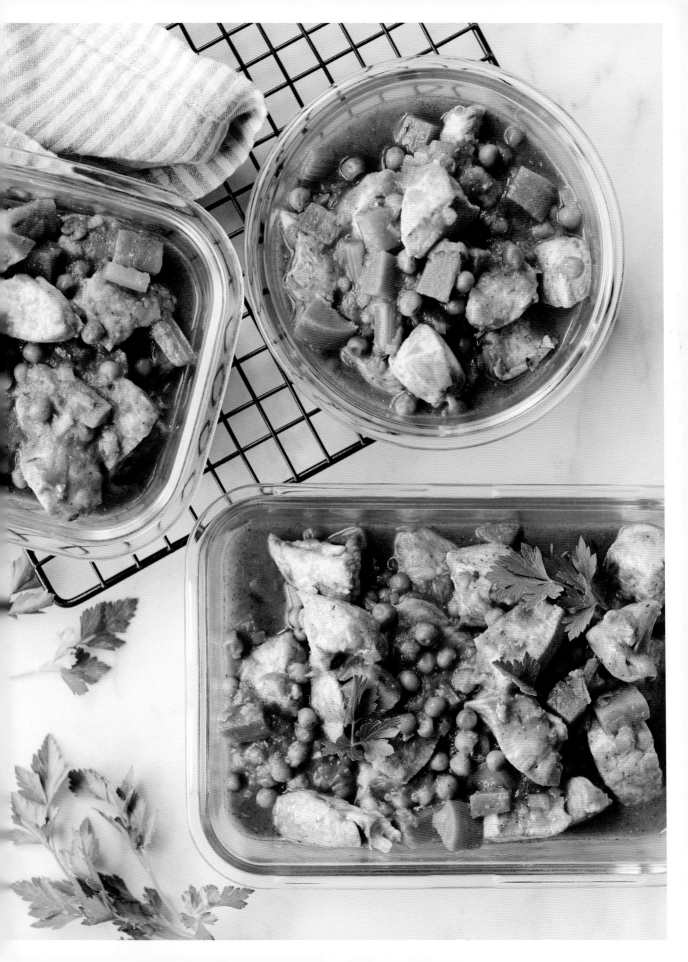

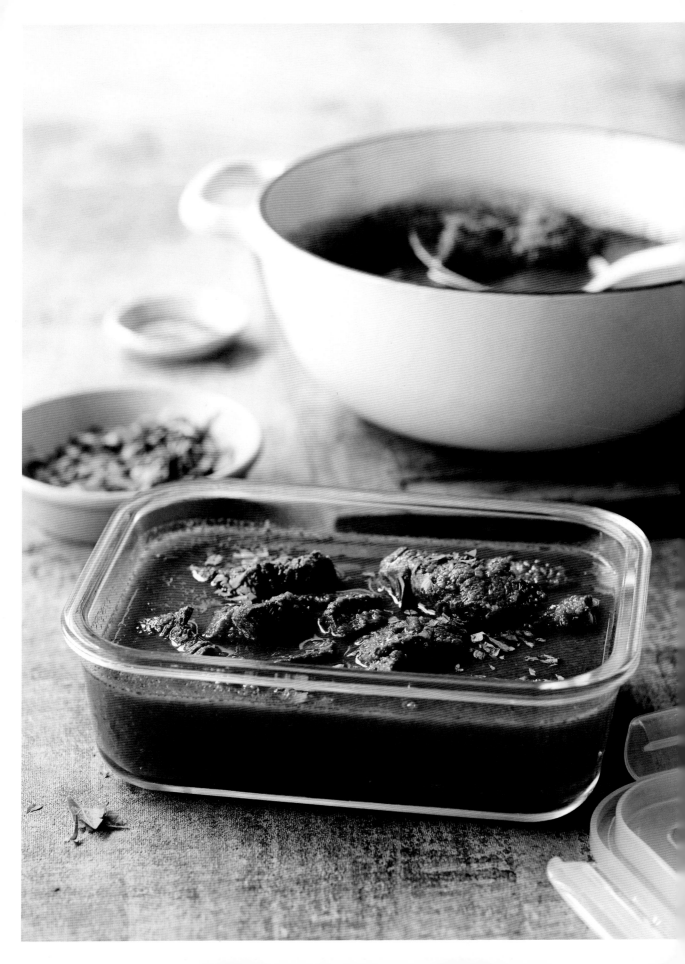

Farmhouse beef ragu

serves 12 (3 x 4-serve meals)
preparation 40 minutes, plus 15 minutes standing time
cooking 2½ hours

80 ml (2½ fl oz/⅓ cup) olive oil
1.8 kg (4 lb) lean gravy beef, cut into 3 cm
 (1¼ inch) pieces
1 litre (35 fl oz/4 cups) beef stock
1 full quantity Farmhouse ragu flavour base (page 131)
15 g (½ oz/½ cup) chopped flat-leaf (Italian) parsley
pasta shapes, rice or mashed potato, to serve

1 Preheat a large heavy-based saucepan over high heat. Place the oil
   and beef in a large bowl, tossing well to combine and coat evenly.

2 Cook the beef in the pan, in six batches, for 5 minutes each until
   almost cooked and light golden. Transfer each batch of beef to a
   large heatproof bowl and reheat the pan until hot before browning
   the next batch.

3 Return all the beef, and any resting juices, to the pan. Add the stock.
   Stir until the mixture just comes to the boil, then reduce the heat
   to medium. Cook, covered and stirring occasionally, for 1½ hours.
   Add the flavour base. Cook, covered and stirring occasionally,
   for 30 minutes or until the beef is falling apart and the sauce has
   thickened slightly.

4 Remove the pan from the heat. Add the parsley and stir to combine.
   Stand, covered, for 15 minutes. Divide the mixture evenly among four
   airtight containers to store.

5 Serve with pasta shapes, rice or mashed potato.

Sweet and sour pork

serves 12 (3 x 4-serve meals)
preparation 45 minutes, plus 15 minutes standing time
cooking 50 minutes

80 ml (2½ fl oz/⅓ cup) macadamia oil
1.8 kg (4 lb) pork fillet, trimmed and
  cut into 2 cm (¾ inch) pieces
185 ml (6 fl oz/¾ cup) chicken stock
1 full quantity Sweet and sour flavour base (page 132)
4 spring onions (scallions), thinly sliced
rice, thin egg noodles or hokkien (egg) noodles, to serve

1 Preheat a large heavy-based saucepan over high heat. Place the oil
  and pork in a large bowl, tossing well to combine and coat evenly.

2 Cook the pork in the pan, in six batches, for 5 minutes each until
  almost cooked and light golden. Transfer each batch of pork to a
  large heatproof bowl and reheat the pan until hot before browning
  the next batch.

3 Return all the pork, and any resting juices, to the pan. Add the stock
  and flavour base. Stir until the mixture just comes to the boil, then
  reduce the heat to medium. Cook, stirring occasionally, for 20 minutes
  or until the pork is cooked and the sauce has thickened slightly.

4 Remove the pan from the heat. Add the spring onion and stir to
  combine. Stand, covered, for 15 minutes. Divide the mixture evenly
  among four airtight containers to store.

5 Serve with rice, thin egg noodles or hokkien (egg) noodles.

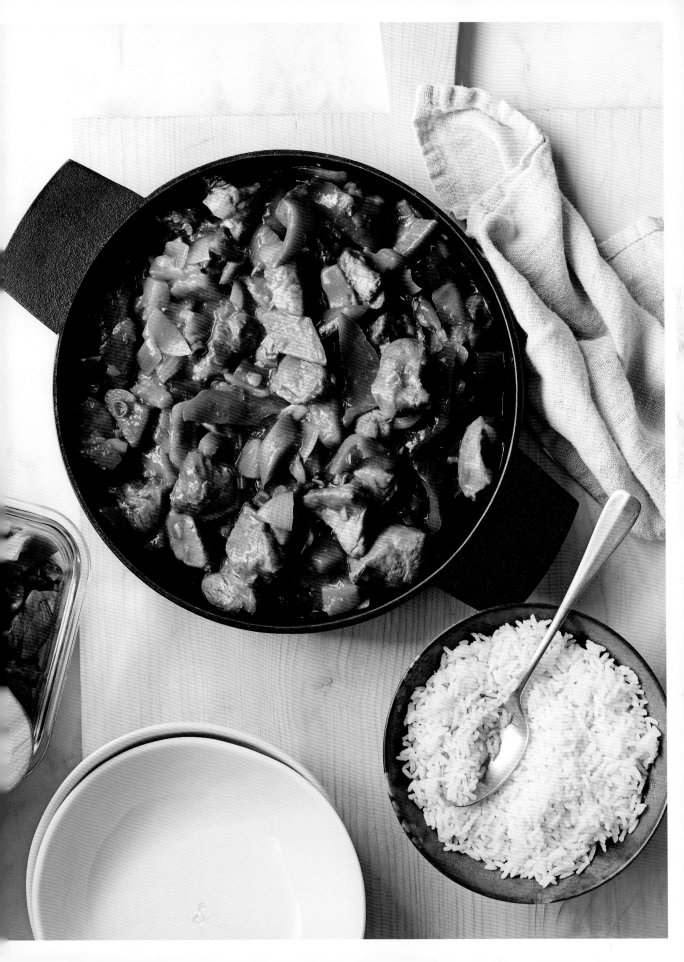

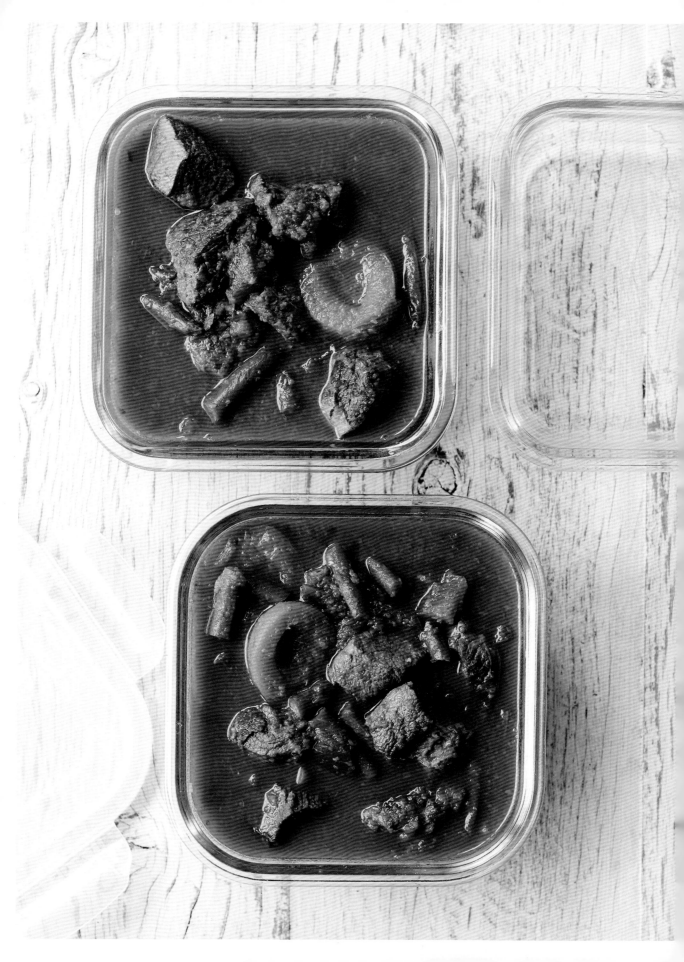

Lamb hotpot

serves 12 (3 x 4-serve meals)
preparation 40 minutes, plus 15 minutes standing time
cooking 2½ hours

80 ml (2½ fl oz/⅓ cup) macadamia oil
1.8 kg (4 lb) lean lamb shoulder,
  cut into 3 cm (1¼ inch) pieces
1 litre (35 fl oz/4 cups) beef stock
400 g (14 oz) tinned chopped tomatoes
1 full quantity Hotpot flavour base (page 132)
pasta shapes, rice, boiled potatoes or mashed potato, to serve

1 Preheat a large heavy-based saucepan over high heat. Place the oil
   and lamb in a large bowl, tossing well to combine and coat evenly.

2 Cook the lamb in the pan, in six batches, for 5 minutes each until
   almost cooked and light golden. Transfer each batch of lamb to a
   large heatproof bowl and reheat the pan until hot before browning
   the next batch.

3 Return all the lamb, and any resting juices, to the pan. Add the stock
   and tomatoes. Stir until the mixture just comes to the boil, then reduce
   the heat to medium. Cook, covered and stirring occasionally, for
   1½ hours. Add the flavour base. Cook, covered and stirring occasionally,
   for 30 minutes or until the lamb is falling apart and the sauce has
   thickened slightly.

4 Stand, covered, for 15 minutes. Divide the mixture evenly among four
   airtight containers to store.

5 Serve with pasta shapes, rice, boiled potatoes or mashed potato.

Honey mustard chicken

serves 12 (3 x 4-serve meals)
preparation 20 minutes, plus 15 minutes standing time
cooking 50 minutes

80 ml (2½ fl oz/⅓ cup) olive oil
1.8 kg (4 lb) chicken tenderloins, trimmed
500 ml (17 fl oz/2 cups) chicken stock
1 full quantity Honey mustard flavour base (page 130)
200 g (7 oz) baby spinach (English spinach) leaves
pasta shapes, rice or mashed potato, to serve

1 Preheat a large heavy-based saucepan over high heat. Place the oil
   and chicken in a large bowl, tossing well to combine and coat evenly.

2 Cook the chicken in the pan, in six batches, for 5 minutes each until
   almost cooked and light golden. Transfer each batch of chicken
   to a large heatproof bowl and reheat the saucepan until hot before
   browning the next batch.

3 Return all the chicken, and any resting juices, to the pan. Add the stock
   and flavour base. Stir until the mixture just comes to the boil, then
   reduce the heat to medium. Cook, stirring occasionally, for 20 minutes
   or until the chicken is cooked and the sauce has thickened slightly.

4 Remove the pan from the heat. Add the spinach and stir to combine.
   Stand, covered, for 15 minutes. Divide the mixture evenly among four
   airtight containers to store.

5 Serve with pasta shapes, rice or mashed potato.

Beef chow mein

serves 12 (3 x 4-serve meals)
preparation 45 minutes, plus 15 minutes standing time
cooking 50 minutes

675 g (1 lb 8 oz) chow mein noodles
boiling water
80 ml (2½ fl oz/⅓ cup) macadamia oil
1.8 kg (4 lb) lean minced (ground) beef
250 ml (9 fl oz/1 cup) beef stock
1 full quantity Chinese chow mein flavour base (page 131)
steamed Asian greens, to serve

1   Soak the noodles in a large bowl of boiling water until they loosen, then drain well.

2   Preheat a large heavy-based saucepan over high heat.

3   Add the oil and beef to the pan. Cook, stirring occasionally and breaking up any lumps with a spoon, for 30 minutes or until cooked and golden.

4   Add the stock and flavour base. Stir until the mixture just comes to the boil, then reduce the heat to medium. Cook, stirring occasionally, for 20 minutes or until the sauce thickens.

5   Remove the pan from the heat. Add the noodles and toss to combine. Stand, covered, for 15 minutes. Divide the mixture evenly among four airtight containers to store.

6   Serve with steamed Asian greens.

Chicken cacciatore

serves 12 (3 x 4-serve meals)
preparation 40 minutes, plus 15 minutes standing time
cooking 2½ hours

80 ml (2½ fl oz/⅓ cup) macadamia oil
1.8 kg (4 lb) skinless chicken thigh fillets,
  trimmed and cut into 3
1 litre (35 fl oz/4 cups) chicken stock
1 full quantity Chicken cacciatore flavour base (page 133)
200 g (7 oz) baby spinach (English spinach) leaves
pasta shapes, rice or mashed potato, to serve

1 Preheat a large heavy-based saucepan over high heat. Place the oil
   and chicken in a large bowl, tossing well to combine and coat evenly.

2 Cook the chicken in the pan, in six batches, for 5 minutes each until
   almost cooked and light golden. Transfer each batch of chicken to a
   large heatproof bowl and reheat the pan until hot before browning the
   next batch.

3 Return all the chicken, and any resting juices, to the pan. Add the stock.
   Stir until the mixture just comes to the boil, then reduce the heat to
   medium. Cook, covered and stirring occasionally, for 1½ hours. Add the
   flavour base. Cook, covered and stirring occasionally, for 30 minutes or
   until the chicken is falling apart and the sauce has thickened slightly.

4 Remove the pan from the heat. Add the spinach and stir to combine.
   Stand, covered, for 15 minutes. Divide the mixture evenly among four
   airtight containers to store.

5 Serve with pasta shapes, rice or mashed potato.

Mild sausage curry

serves 12 (3 x 4-serve meals)
preparation 30 minutes, plus 15 minutes standing time
cooking 40 minutes

80 ml (2½ fl oz/1⅓ cup) macadamia oil
1.8 kg (4 lb) chicken chipolatas
500 ml (17 fl oz/2 cups) chicken stock
1 full quantity Mild coconut curry flavour base (page 133)
410 g (14½ oz) tinned apricot halves in juice
pasta shapes, rice or mashed potato, to serve

1   Preheat a large heavy-based saucepan over high heat. Place the oil
    and chipolatas in a large bowl, tossing well to combine and coat evenly.

2   Cook the chipolatas in the pan, in six batches, for 3 minutes each until
    almost cooked and light golden. Transfer each batch of chipolatas to
    a large heatproof bowl and reheat the pan until hot before browning
    the next batch.

3   Return all the chipolatas, and any resting juices, to the pan. Add the
    stock, flavour base and the apricots and their juice. Stir until the mixture
    just comes to the boil, then reduce the heat to medium. Cook, stirring
    occasionally, for 20 minutes or until the chipolatas are cooked and the
    sauce has thickened slightly.

4   Remove the pan from the heat. Stand, covered, for 15 minutes. Divide
    the mixture evenly among four airtight containers to store.

5   Serve with pasta shapes, rice or mashed potato.

quick & easy sides

Here's your guide to family-favourite sides that are great to have on hand in your pantry, fridge or freezer. Many of these require the simplest preparation or just thawing, and then you can serve them with your selected frozen meal.

HANDY SIDES TO HAVE ON HAND

- Bags of frozen mixed vegetables, which can either be microwaved or quickly blanched
- Shelf-ready packets of cooked rice, which only require microwave heating
- Shelf-ready noodles, which only require a soak in boiling water
- Dried noodles such as rice-stick, rice vermicelli or bean thread, which only require a soak in boiling water
- A couple of large bags of salad mixes from your local supermarket or greengrocers, which can be served as is or easily tossed together with random ingredients from the fridge
- Frozen garlic bread, which can be easily baked in the oven while your meal reheats.

FREEZABLE SIDES TO HAVE ON HAND

RICE

It's important to follow these guidelines for the safe storage and reheating of cooked rice. Cook your favourite rice variety, drain and refresh under cold running tap water until cooled, then drain well again and separate into 2-cup portion packs and freeze for up to 3 months. Defrost in the fridge overnight before microwaving to reheat, or toss in a non-stick frying pan with a little water. Ensure the rice is heated through fully before consuming.

PASTA

Cook your family's favourite pasta variety, then drain and refresh under cold running tap water, making sure to cook for 2 minutes less than the packet directions; then drain well again and separate into 2-cup portion packs and freeze for up to 3 months. Defrost in the fridge overnight before microwaving to reheat, or toss in a non-stick frying pan with a little water.

NOODLES

Soak your family's favourite dried or fresh noodle variety in boiling water or cook in boiling water, then drain and refresh under cold running tap water. Drain well again and separate into 2-cup portion packs and freeze for up to 3 months. Defrost in the fridge overnight before microwaving to reheat, or toss in a non-stick frying pan with a little water.

COUSCOUS

Prepare the couscous according to the packet directions. Using a fork, fluff to separate the grains well, then separate into 2-cup portion packs and freeze for up to 3 months. Defrost in the fridge overnight and serve, or microwave to warm, if desired.

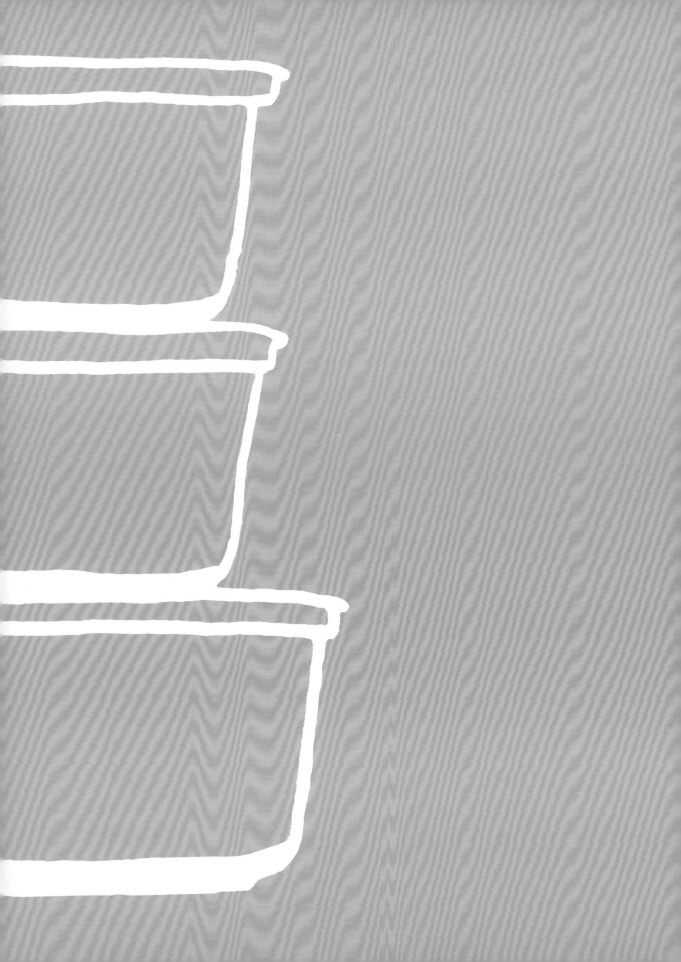

the great make & bake ahead chapter

traybake & take

These traybake and takes are perfect for making ahead in big batches, then transporting and sharing for any occasion, both indoor and outdoor. All recipes use standard non-stick, high-lipped baking trays – 37.5 x 25 x 3 cm (14¾ x 10 x 1¼ inches) – and all make enough to serve 12 people. Simply prep, bake and store these beauties to take along to weekend sports games, picnics and family gatherings, or to serve when people visit and you want to cut down on the post-meal-dishes nightmare. All recipes can be made the day ahead and stored, then served or reheated when you need them.

Each recipe comes with its own personalised prep, storage and transportation tips too – just don't forget to take along some paper napkins, toothpicks or recyclable cutlery, if necessary.

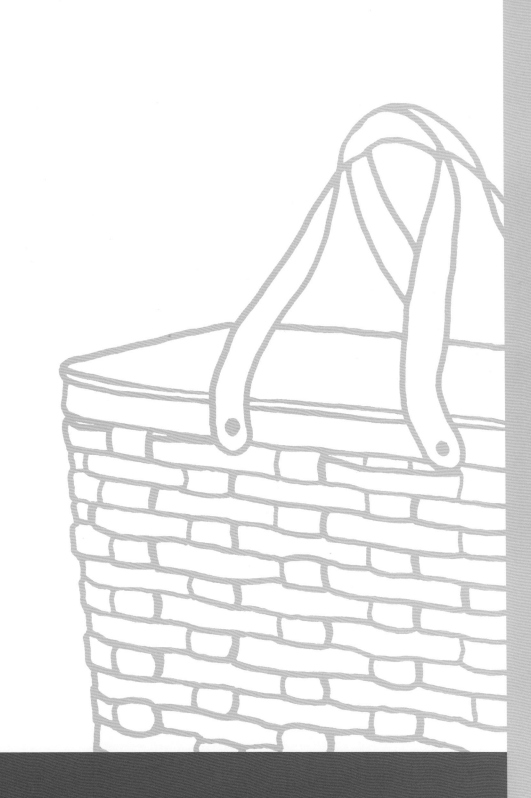

Mini bean tortillas

serves 12 (makes 14)
preparation 45 minutes, plus 15 minutes standing time
cooking 35 minutes

1 red onion, quartered
1 carrot, cut into 2 cm (¾ inch) pieces
200 g (7 oz) store-bought taco sauce
2 tablespoons extra virgin olive oil
400 g (14 oz) tinned red kidney beans, drained and rinsed
250 g (9 oz) store-bought mini stand-and-stuff tortillas
1 corn cob, kernels removed
1 small green capsicum (pepper), finely chopped
2 tablespoons lemon juice
2 tablespoons chopped flat-leaf (Italian) parsley

1 Add the onion and carrot to the mixer bowl, measuring cup in. Chop for 4 sec/speed 5. Scrape down the side of the bowl. Cook for 5 min/120°C/reverse stir/speed 1.

2 Add the taco sauce, oil and beans, measuring cup in. Cook for 10 min/100°C/reverse stir/speed 1.

3 Place all the tortillas, cavity side up, in two 37.5 x 25 x 3 cm (14¾ x 10 x 1¼ inch) non-stick baking trays. Divide the bean mixture evenly among the tortillas.

4 Combine the corn kernels, capsicum, lemon juice and parsley in a bowl.

5 Preheat the oven to 200°C (400°F)/180°C (350°F) fan-forced.

6 Bake the tortillas for 15–20 minutes or until heated and light golden. Stand for 15 minutes, then spoon in the corn mixture and prepare to transport.

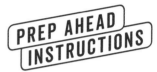

PREP AHEAD INSTRUCTIONS

Make the recipe up to 1 day ahead to the end of step 4. Cool to room temperature, then cover the tray in plastic wrap and place the corn mixture in an airtight container and store both in the fridge. About 45 minutes before transporting, continue with the recipe from step 5.

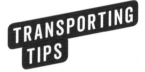

TRANSPORTING TIPS

Cover the tray with a large piece of baking paper, then doubled sheets of foil to enclose tightly. If travelling by car, sit the tray flat in an area where it won't slide around.

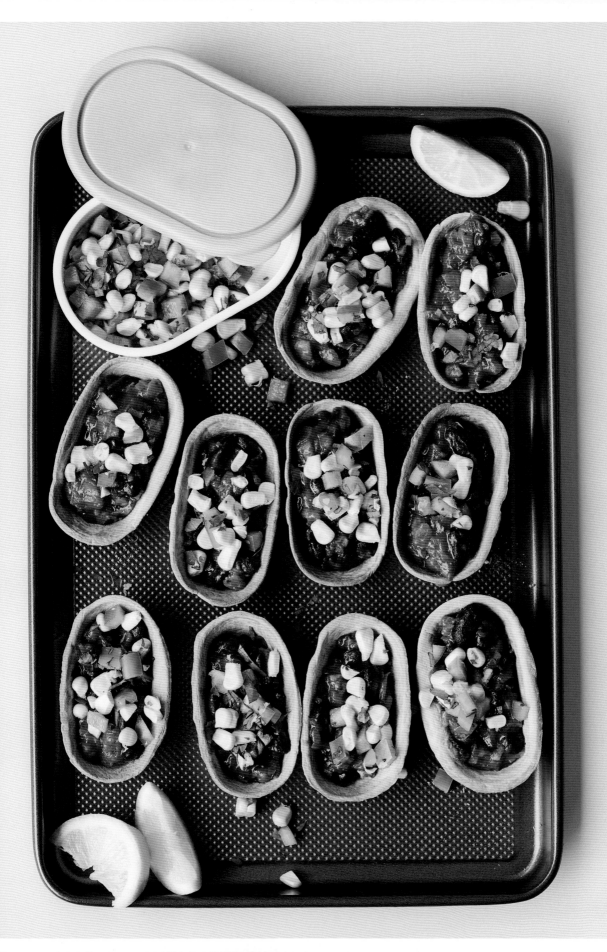

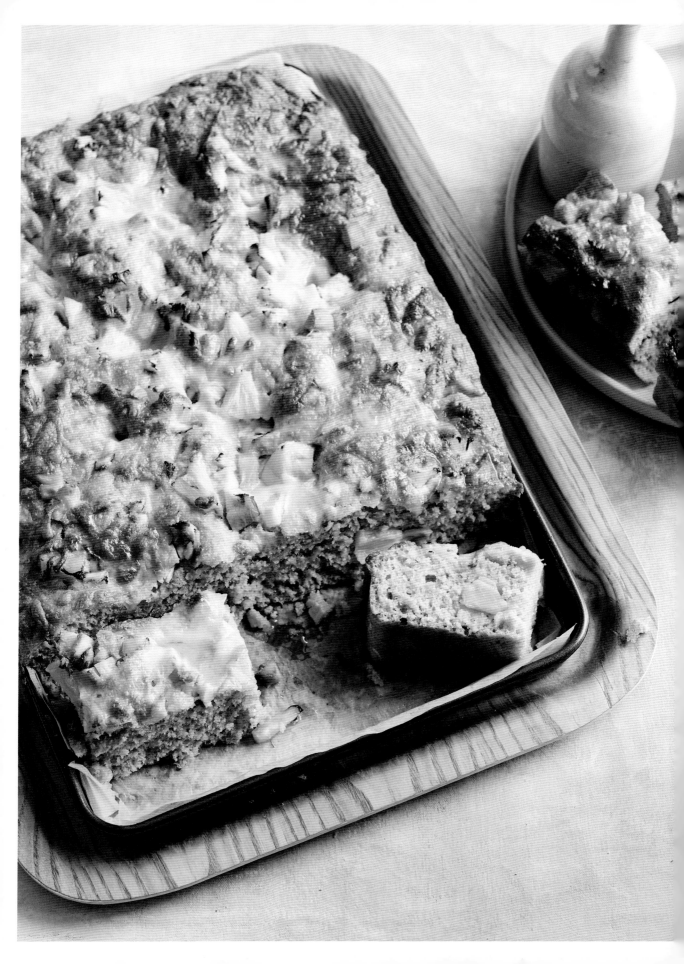

Hawaiian chicken focaccia

serves 12 (makes 24 pieces)
preparation 45 minutes, plus 4 hours proving time,
  plus 15 minutes standing time
cooking 40 minutes

600 g (1 lb 5 oz/4 cups) wholemeal (whole-wheat)
  plain (all-purpose) flour, plus extra for dusting
2 teaspoons sea salt, plus extra for baking
1 tablespoon dried instant yeast
1 teaspoon caster (superfine) sugar
1 tablespoon olive oil, plus 2 tablespoons extra
300 g (10½ oz) barbecued chicken meat, finely chopped
225 g (8 oz) tinned pineapple pieces in juice, drained well and chopped
120 g (4¼ oz/1 cup) grated three-cheese mix (mozzarella, cheddar
  and parmesan)

1 Place the flour and salt in a large bowl. Mix to combine, then make
   a large well in the centre.

2 Add 1 litre (35 fl oz/4 cups) water, the yeast and sugar to the mixer
   bowl, measuring cup in. Warm for 2 min/37°C/speed 1. Pour into the
   well in the flour mixture, then add the oil. Stir to combine – the mixture
   will be runny and sticky. Dust the surface with the extra flour, then cover
   with a piece of baking paper and a clean tea towel (dish towel). Stand
   at room temperature for 2 hours to prove.

3 Line the base and sides of a 37.5 x 25 x 3 cm (14¾ x 10 x 1¼ inch)
   non-stick baking tray with baking paper. Using a flour-dusted hand,
   pull the dough mixture away from the side of the bowl and tip it into
   the prepared tray. Pat out the dough to cover the base of the tray,
   using extra flour if required as the dough will be sticky. Cover with a
   piece of baking paper and a clean tea towel. Stand at room temperature
   for a further 2 hours to prove.

4 Using your fingertips, gently press all over the surface of the dough
   to form indents, then sprinkle evenly with the chicken, pineapple and
   cheese. Gently press the toppings into the dough using your fingertips.

5 Preheat the oven to 220°C (425°F)/200°C (400°F) fan-forced. Sprinkle
   the top of the focaccia with the extra oil. Bake for 35–40 minutes or until
   cooked and golden. Stand for 15 minutes, then cut into pieces in the
   tray before preparing to transport.

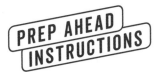

PREP AHEAD INSTRUCTIONS

Make the recipe up to 1 day
ahead to the end of step 4.
Cover the tray with a slightly
damp clean tea towel (dish
towel) – this will help prevent
the dough from drying out –
then wrap in plastic wrap and
store in the fridge. An hour
before transporting, continue
with the recipe from step 5.

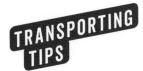

TRANSPORTING TIPS

Cover the tray with a large
piece of baking paper, then
doubled sheets of foil to
enclose tightly. If travelling by
car, sit the tray flat in an area
where it won't slide around.

Minted pea and haloumi bread roll quiches

serves 12 (makes 24 quiches)
preparation 50 minutes, plus 15 minutes standing time
cooking 25 minutes

24 store-bought par-baked white dinner rolls
1 garlic clove
2 tablespoons mint leaves
12 eggs
125 ml (4 fl oz/½ cup) thickened (whipping) cream
180 g (6½ oz) haloumi cheese, finely chopped
65 g (2¼ oz/½ cup) frozen baby peas

1 Preheat the oven to 200°C (400°F)/180°C (350°F) fan-forced. Line the base and sides of two 37.5 x 25 x 3 cm (14¾ x 10 x 1¼ inch) non-stick baking trays with baking paper.

2 Using a small serrated knife, cut a 1 cm (½ inch) thick lid off the top of each dinner roll. Scoop out the soft white bread from inside each roll, leaving a shell. Place the roll shells onto the prepared trays.

3 Add the garlic and mint to the mixer bowl, measuring cup in. Chop for 5 sec/speed 7. Scrape down the side of the bowl.

4 Add the eggs and cream to the mixer bowl, measuring cup in. Mix for 10 sec/speed 4. Scrape down the side of the bowl.

5 Add the haloumi and peas to the mixer bowl, measuring cup in. Combine for 5 sec/reverse stir/speed 3. Spoon the mixture evenly among the bread shells. Place the bread lids on top to enclose.

6 Bake for 20–25 minutes or until the egg has set and the rolls are cooked and golden. Stand for 15 minutes, then prepare for transportation.

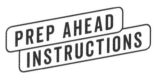

PREP AHEAD INSTRUCTIONS

Make the recipe up to 1 day ahead to the end of step 5. Cover the tray with a slightly damp clean tea towel (dish towel) – this will help prevent the bread from drying out – then wrap in plastic wrap and store in the fridge. An hour before transporting, continue with the recipe from step 6.

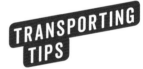

TRANSPORTING TIPS

Cover the tray with a large piece of baking paper, then doubled sheets of foil to enclose tightly. If travelling by car, sit the tray flat in an area where it won't slide around.

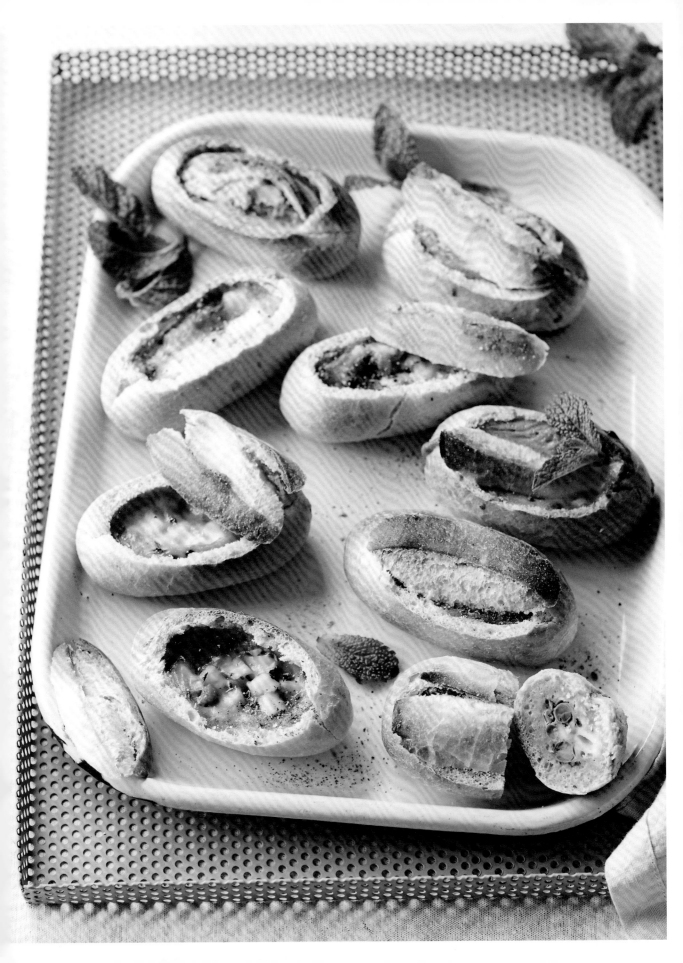

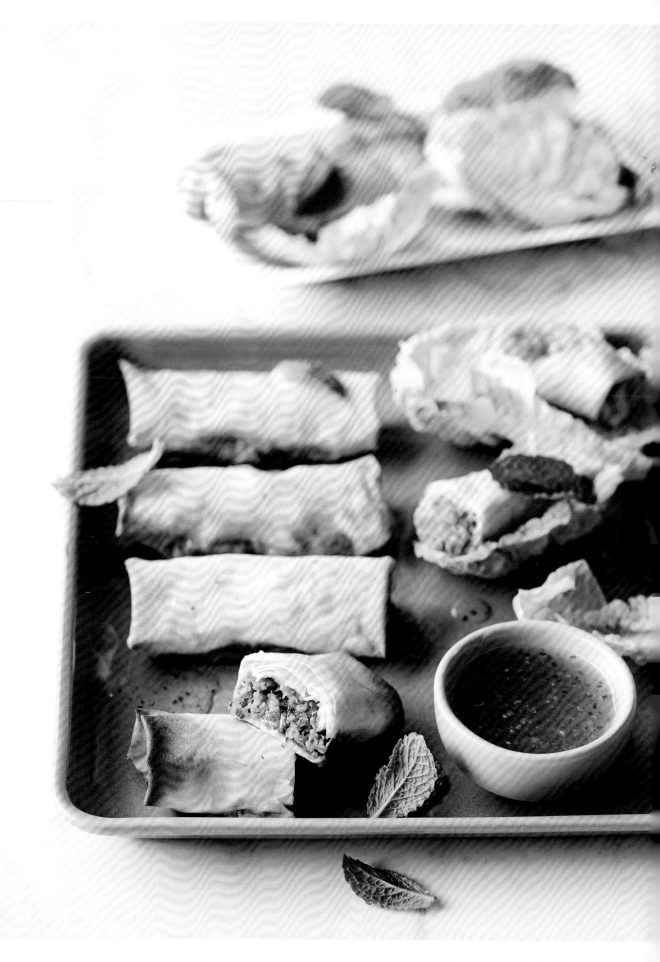

Vegie spring rolls

serves 12 (makes 20 rolls)
preparation 50 minutes, plus 15 minutes cooling time
cooking 30 minutes

1 garlic clove
3 cm (1¼ inch) piece fresh
  ginger, peeled
1 red onion, quartered
2 carrots, cut into 2 cm
  (¾ inch) pieces
225 g (8 oz) tinned water
  chestnuts, drained
330 g (11½ oz/3 cups)
  shredded Chinese cabbage
  (wong bok)
15 g (½ oz/½ cup) coriander
  (cilantro) leaves

2 tablespoons soy sauce
300 g (10½ oz/20 pieces)
  store-bought frozen spring
  roll pastry sheets, at room
  temperature
olive oil cooking spray
baby cos (romaine) lettuce
  leaves, to serve
mint leaves, to serve
store-bought Vietnamese
  dipping sauce, to serve

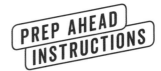

PREP AHEAD INSTRUCTIONS

Make the recipe up to 1 day ahead to the end of step 5, but don't spray with oil. Cool completely, then cover the tray in plastic wrap and store in the fridge. An hour before transporting, spray the rolls with oil and continue with the recipe from step 6.

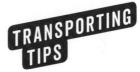

TRANSPORTING TIPS

Cover the tray with a large piece of baking paper, then doubled sheets of foil to enclose tightly. If travelling by car, sit the tray flat in an area where it won't slide around. Place the lettuce, mint and sauce into separate spill-proof, airtight containers and into a chilled portable cooler.

1 Preheat the oven to 220°C (425°F)/200°C (400°F) fan-forced. Line the base and sides of two 37.5 x 25 x 3 cm (14¾ x 10 x 1¼ inch) non-stick baking trays with baking paper.

2 Add the garlic, ginger and onion to the mixer bowl, measuring cup in. Chop for 5 sec/speed 7. Scrape down the side of the bowl. Remove the measuring cup. Cook for 5 min/100°C/speed 2. Transfer the mixture to a bowl.

3 Add the carrot to the mixer bowl, measuring cup in. Chop for 5 sec/speed 7. Scrape down the side of the bowl.

4 Add the water chestnuts, Chinese cabbage, coriander and soy sauce. Combine for 5 sec/speed 5. Transfer to the bowl with the onion mixture, then stir to combine.

5 Separate the spring roll sheets. Place slightly heaped tablespoon measures of the cabbage mixture in the centre of each spring roll sheet. Fold in the edges and wrap up tightly to form a roll, brushing the edges with a little water to seal. Transfer to the prepared trays. Spray both sides of the rolls with oil.

6 Bake for 20–25 minutes, turning occasionally, or until cooked and golden. Cool on the tray for 15 minutes, then prepare for transportation. Serve with baby cos and mint for wrapping the rolls in, and the dipping sauce on the side.

Ratatouille shells

serves 12 (makes 24 filled shells)
preparation 45 minutes, plus 15 minutes standing time
cooking 1 hour

750 g (1 lb 10 oz) jumbo dried
  pasta shells (see note)
1 red onion, quartered
2 garlic cloves
2 tablespoons rosemary leaves
2 tablespoons extra virgin olive oil
400 g (14 oz) tinned chopped tomatoes
1 large zucchini (courgette), finely chopped
1 eggplant (aubergine), finely chopped
1 small red capsicum (pepper), finely chopped
120 g (4¼ oz/1 cup) grated three-cheese mix
  (mozzarella, cheddar and parmesan)

1 Cook the pasta in a large stockpot of boiling water according to the
   packet directions, but minus 2 minutes' cooking time (the pasta will
   keep cooking when grilled). Drain and cool under cold running water.
   Drain well. Transfer the pasta shells to a 37.5 x 25 x 3 cm (14¾ x 10 x
   1¼ inch) non-stick baking tray, cavity side up.

2 Add the onion and garlic to the mixer bowl, measuring cup in. Chop for
   4 sec/speed 5. Scrape down the side of the bowl. Cook for 5 min/120°C/
   reverse stir/speed 1.

3 Add the rosemary, oil and tomatoes, measuring cup removed. Cook for
   12 min/100°C/reverse stir/speed 1. Scrape down the side of the bowl.

4 Add the zucchini, eggplant and capsicum to the mixer bowl, measuring
   cup removed and the steamer basket set over the lid. Cook for 12 min/
   100°C/reverse stir/speed 1.

5 Spoon the eggplant mixture evenly into the cooked pasta shells on
   the tray.

6 Preheat the oven to 220°C (425°F)/200°C (400°F) fan-forced.

7 Sprinkle the cheese evenly on top of each filled pasta shell. Bake
   the pasta for 10–15 minutes or until heated through, the cheese melts
   and the tops are golden. Stand for 15 minutes before preparing
   to transport.

NOTE

You can purchase jumbo dried
pasta shells from supermarkets,
greengrocers and delis. You
can store any remaining
unused shells in an airtight
container in a cool, dark place
for up to 6 months.

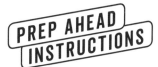

PREP AHEAD
INSTRUCTIONS

Make the recipe up to 1 day
ahead to the end of step 5.
Cool to room temperature, then
cover with a slightly damp clean
tea towel (dish towel) – this will
help prevent the pasta drying
out – then wrap in plastic wrap
and store in the fridge. Half
an hour before transporting,
continue with the recipe from
step 6.

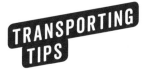

TRANSPORTING
TIPS

Cover the tray with a large
piece of baking paper, then
doubled sheets of foil to
enclose tightly. If travelling by
car, sit the tray flat in an area
where it won't slide around.

Passionfruit custard slice

serves 12 (makes 24 pieces)
preparation 40 minutes, plus cooling time, plus chilling time
cooking 20 minutes

2 sheets frozen butter puff pastry, at room temperature
300 g (10½ oz) unsalted butter, at room temperature
750 g (1 lb 10 oz/6 cups) pure icing (confectioners') sugar
105 g (3½ oz/¾ cup) vanilla custard powder
185 ml (6 fl oz/¾ cup) thickened (whipping) cream
6 passionfruit, seeds and juice scraped (about ½ cup in total)

1 Preheat the oven to 220°C (425°F)/200°C (400°F) fan-forced. Line the
   base and sides of a 37.5 x 25 x 3 cm (14¾ x 10 x 1¼ inch) non-stick
   baking tray with baking paper.

2 Place the pastry sheets, side by side, in the base of the prepared tray,
   trimming them to fit. Place a piece of baking paper over the top, then
   place another baking tray on top. This will allow the pastry to cook but
   without puffing up. Bake for 15–18 minutes or until cooked and golden.
   Cool completely.

3 Add the butter, sugar and custard powder to the mixer bowl, measuring
   cup in. Mix for 10 sec/speed 4. Scrape down the side of the bowl.

4 Add the cream and passionfruit to the mixer bowl, measuring cup in.
   Mix for 5 sec/reverse stir/speed 4. Spread the mixture evenly over the
   pastry in the tray and level the surface. Cover with plastic wrap. Chill
   for 4 hours or overnight until set firm.

5 Using a small, serrated knife, cut the slice into pieces in the tray, then
   prepare for transportation.

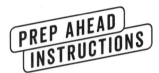

Make the recipe up to
1 day ahead. Cover the tray
in plastic wrap and keep
stored in the fridge.

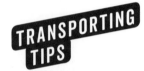

Cover the tray with more
plastic wrap to enclose tightly.
If travelling by car, sit the tray
flat in an area where it won't
slide around.

White choc raspberry blondie

serves 12 (makes 24 pieces)
preparation 40 minutes, plus cooling time
cooking 40 minutes

450 g (1 lb) butter, chopped
500 g (1 lb 2 oz) white chocolate, chopped
330 g (11½ oz/1½ cups) caster (superfine) sugar
8 eggs
335 g (11¾ oz/2¼ cups) plain (all-purpose) flour
65 g (2¼ oz/¾ cup) desiccated coconut
200 g (7 oz) white chocolate baking chips
375 g (13 oz) raspberries

1   Preheat the oven to 180°C (350°F)/160°C (315°F) fan-forced. Line the base and sides of a 37.5 x 25 x 3 cm (14¾ x 10 x 1¼ inch) non-stick baking tray with baking paper.

2   Add the butter and chopped white chocolate to the mixer bowl, measuring cup in. Heat for 5 min/50°C/speed 2 or until melted and smooth. Scrape down the side of the bowl.

3   Add the sugar, eggs, flour and coconut to the mixer bowl, measuring cup in. Mix for 20 sec/speed 5. Scrape down the side of the bowl.

4   Spoon the mixture into the prepared tray and level the surface. Sprinkle the top evenly with the white chocolate chips and raspberries. Bake for 30–35 minutes, or until just cooked and golden. Cool completely in the tray. Cut into pieces in the tray, then prepare for transportation.

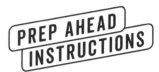

PREP AHEAD INSTRUCTIONS

Make the recipe up to 1 day ahead. Cool completely, then cover the tray in plastic wrap and store in a cool, dark place.

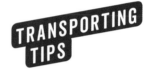

TRANSPORTING TIPS

Cover the tray with more plastic wrap to enclose tightly. If travelling by car, sit the tray flat in an area where it won't slide around.

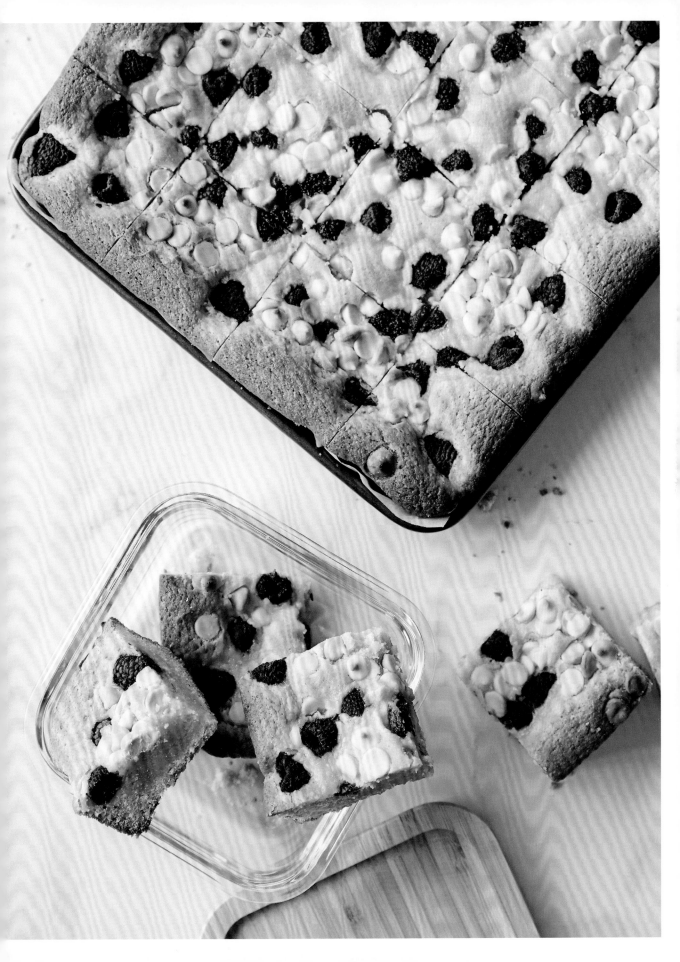

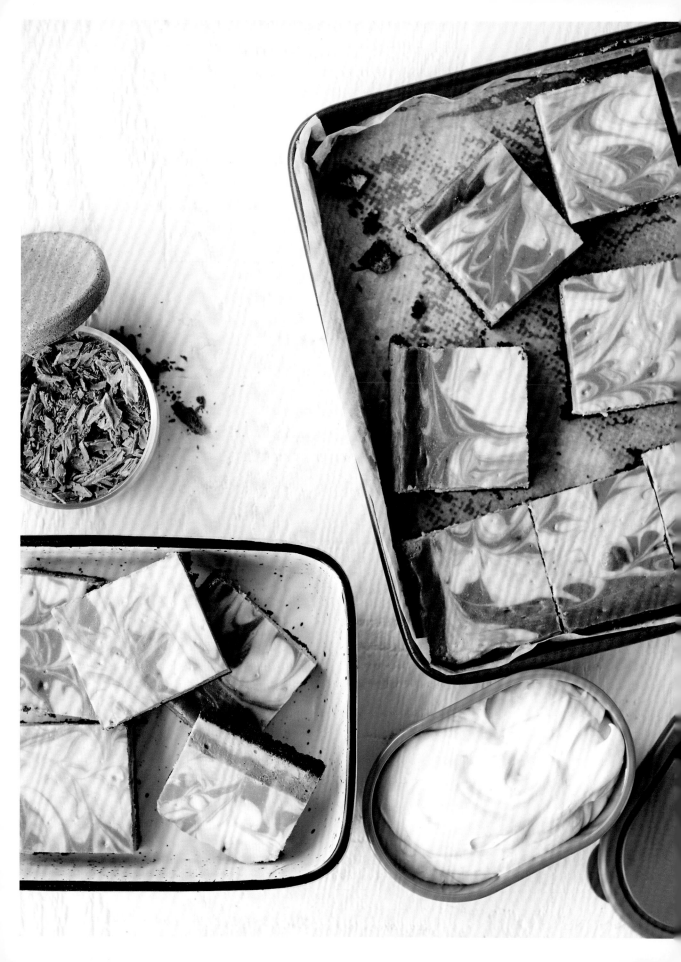

Tiramisu baked cheesecake

serves 12 (makes 24 pieces)
preparation 45 minutes, plus chilling, plus cooling time
cooking 45 minutes

200 g (7 oz) unsalted butter
500 g (1 lb 2 oz) chocolate
  ripple cookies, broken in half
75 g (2½ oz/⅓ cup) caster
  (superfine) sugar
5 eggs, at room temperature
2 teaspoons pure vanilla extract
1 kg (2 lb 4 oz) cream cheese,
  at room temperature

450 g (1 lb) sour cream,
  at room temperature
2 tablespoons decaffeinated
  instant coffee granules
2 tablespoons sweetened
  drinking chocolate powder
125 g (4½ oz/⅔ cup) brown sugar
whipped cream, to serve
crumbled Flake bars, to serve

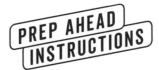

PREP AHEAD INSTRUCTIONS

Make the recipe up to
2 days ahead. Cover the tray
in plastic wrap and keep
stored in the fridge.

TRANSPORTING TIPS

Cover the tray with more
plastic wrap to enclose tightly.
If travelling by car, sit the
tray flat in an area where it
won't slide around. Place the
whipped cream and chocolate
into separate spill-proof, airtight
containers, then into a chilled
portable cooler.

1 Line the base and sides of a 37.5 x 25 x 3 cm (14¾ x 10 x 1¼ inch)
   non-stick baking tray with baking paper.

2 Chop the butter and add it to the mixer bowl, measuring cup in. Melt
   for 2 min/100°C/speed 2. Scrape down the side of the bowl. Add the
   cookies, measuring cup in. Mix for 5 sec/speed 7 or until finely crushed.
   Transfer the mixture to the prepared tray, pressing down firmly to cover
   the base evenly. Chill for 20 minutes or until firm. Clean the mixer bowl.
   Preheat the oven to 160°C (315°F)/140°C (275°F) fan-forced.

3 Add the caster sugar, 2 of the eggs, the vanilla, 375 g (13 oz) of the
   cream cheese and 150 g (5½ oz) of the sour cream to the mixer bowl.
   Mix for 30 sec/speed 7, or until well combined. Transfer the runny
   mixture to a bowl. Clean the mixer bowl.

4 Add the coffee, chocolate powder and 1 tablespoon water to the mixer
   bowl, measuring cup in. Cook for 1 min/100°C/speed 2 or until dissolved.

5 Add the brown sugar, the remaining eggs, cream cheese and sour
   cream to the mixer bowl, measuring cup in. Mix for 30 sec/speed 7.
   Dollop the mixture over the cookie base, then drizzle with the white
   cheese mixture and level the surface. Use the tip of a skewer to run
   through both mixtures to create a marbled effect.

6 Bake for 40 minutes or until firm to the touch around the edges, with
   a slight wobble in the centre. Turn the oven off. Leave the cheesecake
   in the oven to cool completely, with the door 20 cm (8 inches) ajar.

7 Transfer the cooled cheesecake to the fridge and chill for 4 hours or
   overnight. Cut into pieces in the tray, then prepare for transportation.

Double-choc cookie brownie

serves 12 (makes 24 pieces)
preparation 40 minutes, plus cooling time
cooking 30 minutes

400 g (14 oz) butter, chopped
400 g (14 oz) dark chocolate melts (buttons)
285 g (10 oz/1½ cups) brown sugar
6 eggs, at room temperature
40 g (1½ oz/⅓ cup) unsweetened cocoa powder
180 g (6½ oz/1½ cups) gluten-free plain
  (all-purpose) flour
230 g (8½ oz) mini chocolate Oreo cookies, broken in half

1 Preheat the oven to 180°C (350°F)/160°C (315°F) fan-forced. Line the base and sides of a 37.5 x 25 x 3 cm (14¾ x 10 x 1¼ inch) non-stick baking tray with baking paper.

2 Add the butter and chocolate to the mixer bowl, measuring cup in. Heat for 5 min/50°C/speed 2 or until melted and smooth. Scrape down the side of the bowl.

3 Add the sugar to the mixer bowl, measuring cup in. Mix for 10 sec/ speed 3. Scrape down the side of the bowl.

4 Add the eggs, cocoa and flour to the mixer bowl, measuring cup in. Mix for 5 sec/speed 4. Scrape down the side of the bowl. Mix for 5 sec/speed 4. Scrape down the side of the bowl.

5 Add the cookies to the mixer bowl, measuring cup in. Combine for 10 sec/reverse stir/speed 2. Transfer the mixture to the prepared tray and level the surface.

6 Bake the brownie for 20–25 minutes or until just set in the centre. Cool completely in the tray. Cut into pieces in the tray, then prepare for transportation.

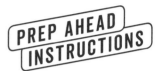

PREP AHEAD INSTRUCTIONS

Make the recipe up to 2 days ahead. Cover the tray in plastic wrap and keep stored in the fridge.

TRANSPORTING TIPS

Cover the tray with more plastic wrap to enclose tightly. If travelling by car, sit the tray flat in an area where it won't slide around.

Cheat's lemon meringue

serves 12 (makes 20 pieces)
preparation 45 minutes, plus cooling time,
  plus chilling time
cooking 35 minutes

225 g (8 oz) unsalted butter, at room temperature
220 g (7¾ oz/½ cup) caster (superfine) sugar
2 teaspoons pure vanilla extract
375 g (13 oz/2½ cups) plain (all-purpose) flour
170 ml (5½ fl oz/⅔ cup) strained fresh lemon juice (see note)
70 g (2½ oz/½ cup) vanilla custard powder
4 eggs
800 ml (28 fl oz) thin (pouring/whipping) cream
200 g (7 oz) store-bought vanilla mini meringues

1 Preheat the oven to 180°C (350°F)/160°C (315°F) fan-forced. Line the base and sides of a 37.5 x 25 x 3 cm (14¾ x 10 x 1¼ inch) non-stick baking tray with baking paper.

2 Add the butter and half the sugar to the mixer bowl, measuring cup in. Mix for 20 sec/speed 5. Scrape down the side of the bowl.

3 Add the vanilla and flour to the mixer bowl, measuring cup in. Mix for 20 sec/speed 4. Scrape down the side of the bowl. Mix for 20 sec/speed 4. Transfer the mixture to the prepared tray. Using slightly damp fingertips, press down firmly to cover the base evenly. Bake for 20–25 minutes or until light golden. Cool completely in the tray. Clean the mixer bowl.

4 Add the lemon juice, custard powder, eggs, cream and the remaining sugar to the mixer bowl, measuring cup in. Mix for 45 sec/speed 2. Scrape down the side of the bowl. Cook for 7 min/80°C/speed 2 until slightly thickened. Pour the lemon mixture over the base in the tray and level the surface. Cool to room temperature, then transfer to the fridge. Chill for 4 hours or overnight until set firm.

5 Arrange the meringues on top of the lemon filling in the tray. Cut into pieces in the tray, then prepare for transportation.

NOTE

You will need 4 large lemons for the juice.

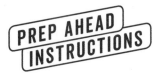

PREP AHEAD INSTRUCTIONS

Make the recipe up to 1 day ahead to the end of step 4. Cover the tray in plastic wrap and keep stored in the fridge.

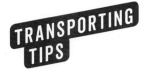

TRANSPORTING TIPS

About 15 minutes before transporting, arrange the mini meringues on top. Cover the tray with more plastic wrap to enclose tightly. If travelling by car, sit the tray flat in an area where it won't slide around.

Funfetti ripple cake

serves 12 (makes 24 pieces)
preparation 50 minutes, plus cooling time, plus 1 hour chilling time
cooking 50 minutes

250 g (9 oz) butter, at room temperature
330 g (11½ oz/1½ cups) white sugar
600 g (1 lb 5 oz/4 cups) self-raising flour
375 ml (13 fl oz/1½ cups) milk
3 teaspoons pure vanilla extract
4 eggs
150 g (5½ oz/1 cup) rainbow sprinkles
blue, red, yellow and green food colouring

BUTTERCREAM
360 g (12¾ oz/3 cups) icing (confectioners') sugar mixture, sifted
250 g (9 oz) unsalted butter, at room temperature
2 tablespoons milk of choice
blue and green food colouring

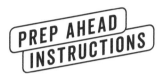

PREP AHEAD INSTRUCTIONS

Make the recipe up to 2 days ahead. Cover the tray in plastic wrap and keep stored in the fridge.

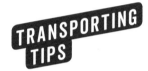

TRANSPORTING TIPS

Cover the tray with more plastic wrap to enclose tightly. If travelling by car, sit the tray flat in an area where it won't slide around.

1 Preheat the oven to 160°C (315°F)/140°C (275°F) fan-forced. Line the base and sides of a 37.5 x 25 x 3 cm (14¾ x 10 x 1¼ inch) non-stick baking tray with baking paper.

2 Add the butter, sugar, flour, milk and vanilla to the mixer bowl, measuring cup in. Mix for 1 min 30 sec/speed 4. Scrape down the side of the bowl. Mix for 1 min 30 sec/speed 4. Scrape down the side of the bowl. Add the eggs, measuring cup in. Mix for 10 sec/speed 6.

3 Add half the sprinkles to the mixer bowl, measuring cup in. Mix for 3 sec/speed 5. Divide the mixture evenly into three separate bowls. Tint one bowl purple by adding 6 drops of blue and 9 drops of red food colouring and stir to combine. Tint another bowl lime green by adding 5 drops of yellow and 10 drops of green food colouring and stir to combine. Tint the last bowl aqua by adding 8 drops of blue and 2 drops of green food colouring and stir to combine. Dollop the tinted batters all over the base of the prepared tray. Use a skewer to swirl them together to create a marbled effect. Bake the cake for 45–50 minutes or until a skewer inserted in the centre comes out clean and the top is light golden. Cool completely in the tray.

4 Make the buttercream by adding the icing sugar and butter to the mixer bowl, measuring cup in. Mix for 10 sec/speed 6. Scrape down the side of the bowl. Insert the butterfly whisk. Add the milk to the mixer bowl. Whisk for 2 min/speed 3. Add 3 drops of blue and 1 drop of green food colouring to the mixer bowl, measuring cup in. Whisk for 30 sec/speed 3.

5 Spread the buttercream over the cooled cake. Decorate with the remaining sprinkles. Chill for 1 hour or until the buttercream is firm. Cut into pieces in the tray, then prepare for transportation.

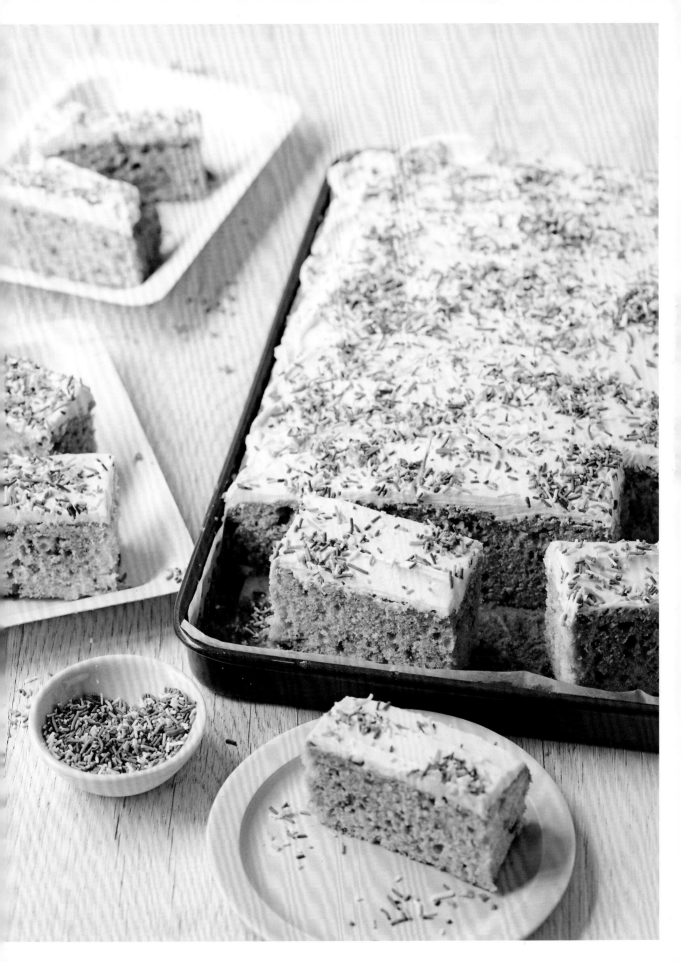

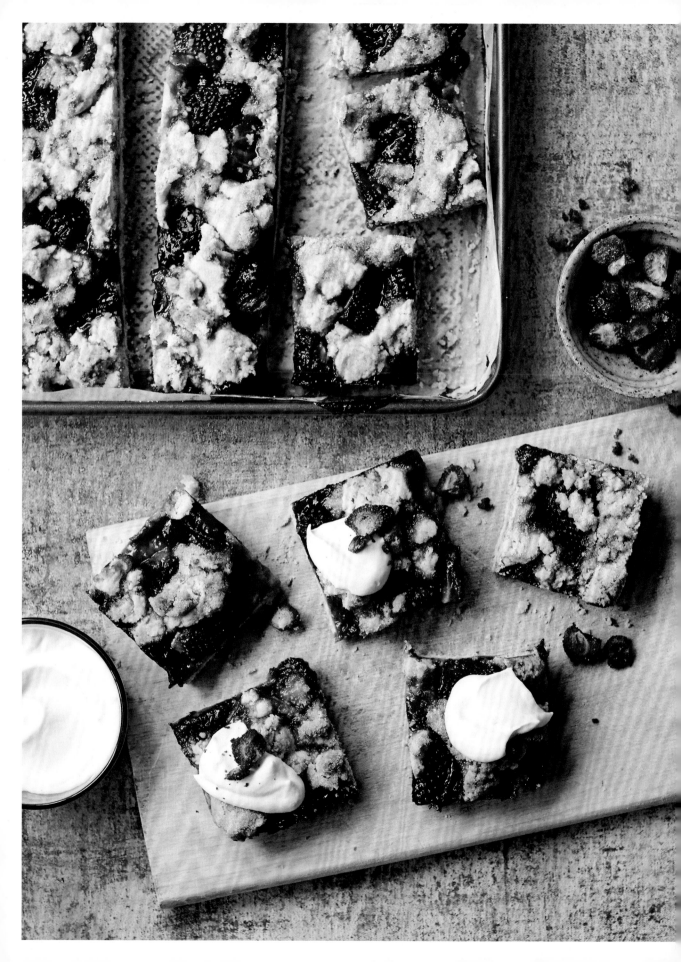

Strawberry shortcake

serves 12 (makes 24 pieces)
preparation 45 minutes, plus 10 minutes freezing time,
  plus cooling time
cooking 40 minutes

250 g (9 oz) butter, chopped
110 g (3¾ oz/½ cup) caster (superfine) sugar,
  plus 75 g (2½ oz/⅓ cup) extra for sprinkling
300 g (10½ oz/2 cups) self-raising flour
300 g (10½ oz/2 cups) plain (all-purpose) flour,
  plus extra for dusting
2 eggs
320 g (11¼ oz/½ cup) smooth strawberry jam
3 teaspoons pure vanilla extract
500 g (1 lb 2 oz) strawberries, hulled and halved
vanilla whipped cream, to serve (see note)
dehydrated strawberries, to serve

1 Line the base and sides of a 37.5 x 25 x 3 cm (14¾ x 10 x 1¼ inch) non-stick baking tray with baking paper.

2 Add the butter and sugar to the mixer bowl, measuring cup in. Chop for 3 sec/speed 6. Scrape down the side of the bowl.

3 Add the flours and eggs to the mixer bowl, measuring cup in. Knead for 1 min 30 sec/kneading mode or until well combined. The mixture will be crumbly. Transfer to a lightly floured surface, then divide into two equal portions. Press one portion of the dough firmly and evenly over the base of the tray. Freeze for 10 minutes.

4 Preheat the oven to 180°C (350°F)/160°C (315°F) fan-forced.

5 Clean the mixer bowl. Add the jam and 2 tablespoons water to the mixer bowl, measuring cup in. Cook for 3 min/60°C/speed 1.

6 Add the vanilla extract and strawberries to the mixer bowl, measuring cup in. Mix for 1 min/reverse stir/speed 2. Spread the mixture evenly over the dough in the base of the prepared tray. Crumble the remaining portion of dough over. Sprinkle evenly with the extra sugar.

7 Bake for 30–35 minutes or until golden. Cool completely in the tray. Cut the shortcake into pieces in the tray, then prepare for transportation.

NOTE

Make vanilla whipped cream by adding 300 ml (10½ fl oz) thin (pouring/whipping) cream and 2 teaspoons pure vanilla extract to the mixer bowl. Insert the butterfly whisk. Whisk for 3 sec/speed 3 or until soft peaks form. Transfer to a spill-proof, airtight container and keep chilled until transporting.

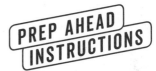

PREP AHEAD INSTRUCTIONS

Make the recipe up to 1 day ahead. Cool completely, then cover the tray in plastic wrap and store in a cool, dark place.

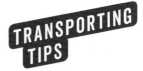

TRANSPORTING TIPS

Cover the tray with more plastic wrap to enclose tightly. If travelling by car, sit the tray flat in an area where it won't slide around. Place the cream and dehydrated strawberries into separate spill-proof, airtight containers and into a chilled portable cooler.

bake & store

Whether it's something special, a simple weekend treat or a snack on the go, this chapter has it all. These sweet and savoury baked favourites can be made ahead and will store well in your pantry, fridge or freezer. The recipes are great for simple grab-and-go lunchbox fillers, for Saturday sports snacking, Sunday brunch or afternoon sweet treats to simply enjoy with a hot cuppa. In every which way, these beauties will satisfy every tastebud requirement in your household, as there's something for everyone. Detailed storage information is provided for all recipes.

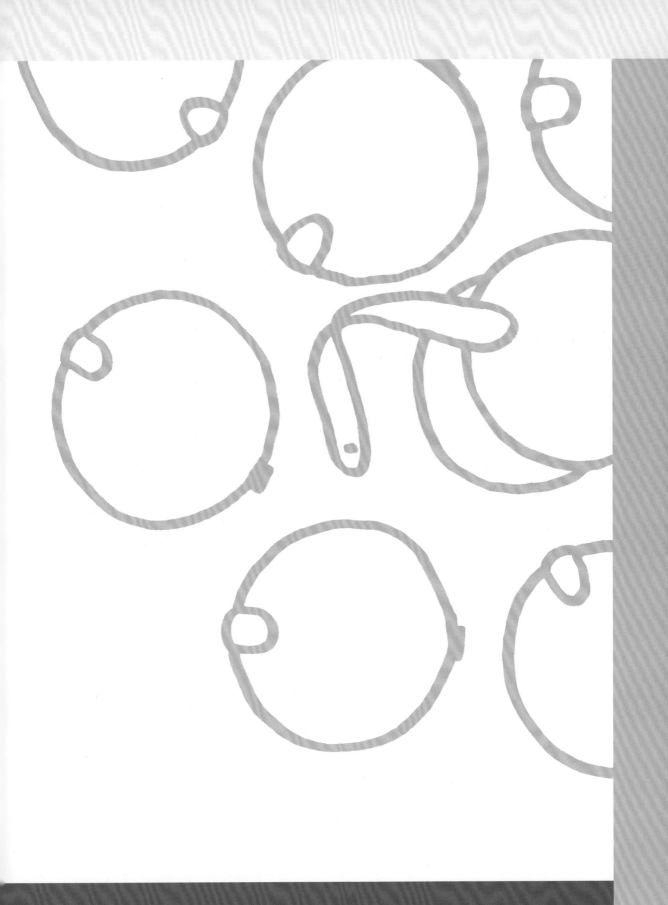

Spinach and feta gozleme

makes 24
preparation 50 minutes, plus 30 minutes proving time
cooking 1 hour 15 minutes

2 tablespoons instant dried yeast
2 teaspoons caster (superfine) sugar
900 g (2 lb/6 cups) plain, strong bread and pizza flour, plus extra for dusting
80 ml (2½ fl oz/⅓ cup) olive oil
2 garlic cloves
10 g (¼ oz/½ cup) flat-leaf (Italian) parsley leaves

5 g (⅛ oz/¼ cup) mint leaves
200 g (7 oz) baby spinach (English spinach) leaves
500 g (1 lb 2 oz) Greek feta cheese, crumbled
freshly ground black pepper
olive oil cooking spray
lemon wedges, to serve

STORAGE

The gozleme can be prepared up to the end of step 3, then frozen in small stacks, sandwiched between sheets of baking paper, then placed in freezer-safe bags for up to 2 months. Bake from frozen, and sprayed with oil on both sides, at 220°C (425°F)/200°C (400°F) fan-forced, for 15–20 minutes or until cooked and golden. Store the cooked, cooled gozleme in between sheets of baking paper in an airtight container in the fridge for up to 3 days.

1 Add 600 ml (21 fl oz) water, the yeast and sugar to the mixer bowl, measuring cup in. Heat for 3 min/50°C/speed 2. Scrape down the side of the bowl. Add the flour and oil to the mixer bowl, measuring cup in. Knead for 2 min/kneading mode. Transfer the dough to a lightly floured bowl, cover and stand in a warm place for 30 minutes to prove. Clean the mixer bowl.

2 While the dough is proving, add the garlic, parsley, mint and spinach to the mixer bowl, measuring cup in. Chop for 2 sec/speed 6, or until finely chopped. Transfer to a bowl. Add the feta and stir to combine. Season with pepper.

3 Divide the dough into 24 equal portions. Roll each portion out on a lightly floured work surface to a large 20 cm (8 inch) wide circle. Add 2 slightly heaped tablespoons of the spinach mixture onto one half of the dough, leaving a 1 cm (½ inch) border. Fold over the dough to enclose the spinach, flattening the parcel slightly in the palm of your hand to remove any air bubbles, then pinching the edges together tightly to seal.

4 Place two large non-stick frying pans over medium–high heat. Spray them liberally with oil. Add one gozleme at a time to each pan. Cook, in batches, for 2–3 minutes, then spray the uncooked side liberally with oil and flip. Cook for a further 2–3 minutes or until cooked and golden. Transfer to a heatproof plate and cover loosely with foil to keep warm. Repeat with the remaining gozleme, using more oil with each one. Serve warm with the lemon wedges, or cool completely, then store.

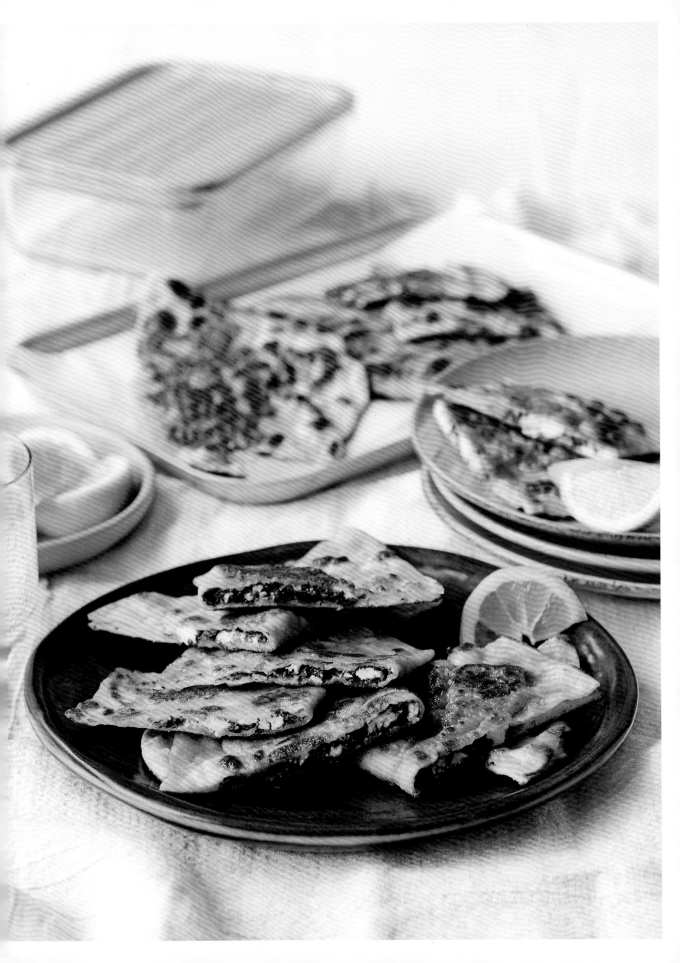

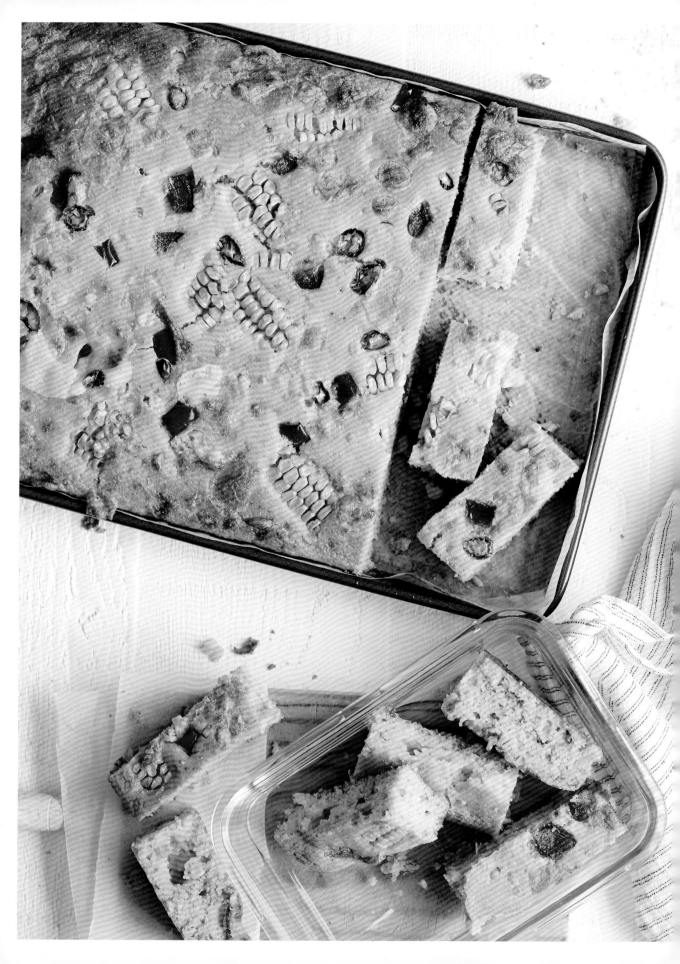

Loaded cornbread

serves 12 (makes 24 pieces)
preparation 45 minutes, plus 10 minutes cooling time
cooking 30 minutes

380 g (13½ oz/2 cups) instant polenta
300 g (10½ oz/2 cups) self-raising flour
2 teaspoons baking powder
75 g (2½ oz/⅓ cup) caster (superfine) sugar
80 g (2¾ oz) butter
500 ml (17 fl oz/2 cups) buttermilk
4 eggs
2 corn cobs, kernels removed
1 red capsicum (pepper), finely chopped
2 long green chillies, thinly sliced
235 g (8½ oz) sharp, soft and crumbly cheddar
   cheese, crumbled

1 Preheat the oven to 200°C (400°F)/180°C (350°F) fan-forced. Line
   a 37.5 x 25 x 3 cm (14¾ x 10 x 1¼ inch) non-stick baking tray with
   baking paper.

2 Add the polenta, flour, baking powder and sugar to the mixer bowl,
   measuring cup in. Mix for 5 sec/speed 4. Transfer to a bowl.

3 Add the butter to the mixer bowl, measuring cup in. Melt for
   1 min/100°C/speed 2.

4 Add the buttermilk and eggs to the mixer bowl, measuring cup in.
   Mix for 5 sec/speed 4.

5 Add the reserved polenta mixture to the mixer bowl, measuring cup in.
   Mix for 10 sec/speed 4. Scrape down the side of the bowl.

6 Add the corn kernels, capsicum, chillies and cheddar to the mixer bowl,
   measuring cup in. Mix for 10 sec/reverse stir/speed 2. Transfer the
   mixture to the prepared tray.

7 Bake the cornbread for 25–30 minutes or until a skewer inserted in the
   centre comes out clean and the top is golden. Stand on the tray for
   10 minutes to cool, then serve warm, or cool completely and store.

This cornbread is delicious
served with lashings of butter
and alongside your favourite
beef or bean chilli, soup,
casserole or stew, used as
a breakfast bread, or added
to any barbecue meal.

The cooked cornbread
can be stored in an airtight
container in the fridge for up
to 5 days or separated into
portions and placed in freezer-
safe bags, then frozen for up
to 3 months. Defrost in the
fridge overnight, then either
reheat in the oven or split in half
and either toast under a grill
(broiler) or cook in a chargrill
pan or on the barbecue.

Margherita pizza bites

makes 24
preparation 1 hour, plus 1 hour proving time,
  plus 3 minutes standing time
cooking 10 minutes

375 ml (13 fl oz/1½ cups) lukewarm water
1 tablespoon instant dried yeast
2 teaspoons caster (superfine) sugar
450 g (1 lb/3 cups) plain, strong bread
  and pizza flour, plus extra for dusting
1 tablespoon sea salt
60 ml (2 fl oz/¼ cup) extra virgin olive oil,
  plus extra to drizzle
olive oil cooking spray
140 g (5 oz/½ cup) pizza sauce with garlic,
  onion and herbs
24 large basil leaves
12 cherry tomatoes, halved
24 mini cherry bocconcini (fresh baby
  mozzarella cheese)
parmesan cheese shavings, to serve

STORAGE

The cooked pizza bites can be
stored in an airtight container
in the fridge for up to 3 days
or separated into portions and
placed in freezer-safe bags
and frozen for up to 3 months.
Defrost in the fridge overnight,
then reheat in the oven.

1 Add the water, yeast and sugar to the mixer bowl, measuring cup in.
   Heat for 3 min/50°C/speed 2. Scrape down the side of the bowl.

2 Add the flour, salt and oil to the mixer bowl, measuring cup in. Knead
   for 2 min/kneading mode. Transfer to a lightly floured bowl. Cover and
   stand in a warm place to prove for 1 hour or until doubled in size.

3 Preheat the oven to 240°C (475°F)/220°C (425°F) fan-forced. Grease two
   12-hole, 1½ tablespoon capacity round-based patty pans with the oil.

4 Divide the dough into 24 equal portions then, using lightly floured
   hands, flatten into 8 cm (3¼ inch) rounds. Place the rounds into the
   prepared pans, pressing down firmly to mould into the holes. Spoon the
   pizza sauce evenly into the centres of the dough, then top with a basil
   leaf, then a cherry tomato half, then a cherry bocconcini.

5 Bake for 8–10 minutes, swapping the pans around on the oven
   shelves halfway through baking, or until the pizza bites are cooked
   and golden. Drizzle the tops with the extra oil and sprinkle with the
   parmesan. Stand in the pans for 3 minutes, then transfer to a wire
   rack. Serve warm or cool completely, then store.

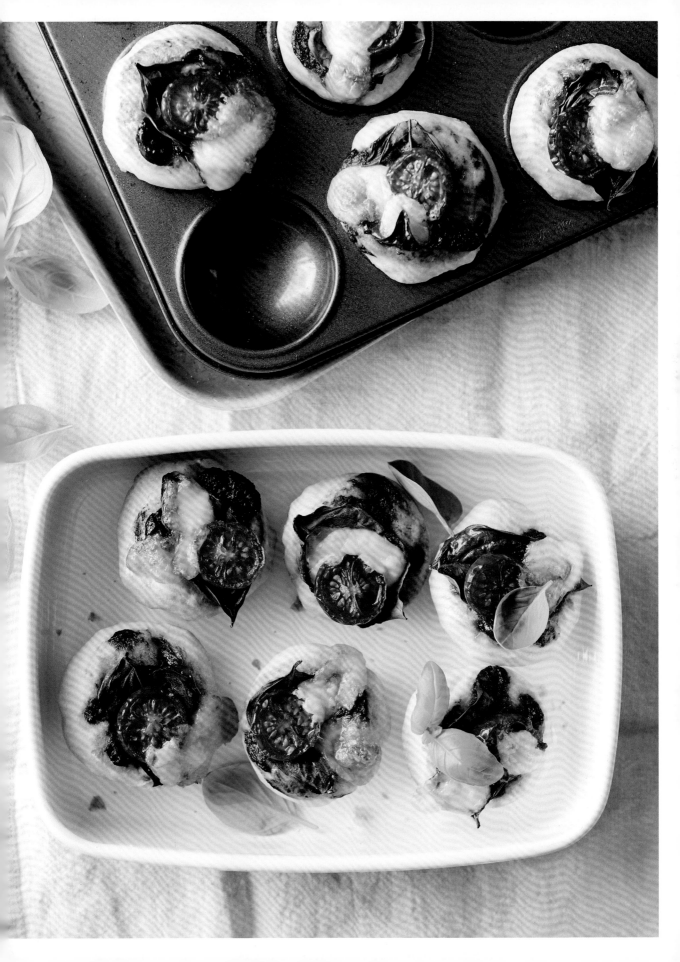

Chorizo loaf

makes 2 loaves (serves 16)
preparation 45 minutes, plus 5 minutes standing time,
 plus cooling time
cooking 50 minutes

200 ml (7 fl oz) olive oil,
 plus extra for greasing
6 eggs
200 ml (7 fl oz) milk of choice
200 g (7 oz) semi-dried
 (sun-blushed) tomatoes
200 g (7 oz) diced chorizo

375 g (13 oz/2½ cups)
 self-raising flour
4 spring onions (scallions),
 thinly sliced
200 g (7 oz) grated provolone
 cheese
sea salt flakes
freshly ground black pepper

1 Preheat the oven to 180°C (350°F)/160°C (315°F) fan-forced. Grease and line the base only of two 22 x 10 x 7 cm (8½ x 4 x 2¾ inch) loaf (bar) tins.

2 Add the oil, eggs, milk, tomatoes and chorizo to the mixer bowl, measuring cup in. Mix for 25 sec/speed 6. Scrape down the side of the bowl.

3 Add the flour, spring onion and provolone. Combine for 10 sec/reverse stir/speed 5. Scrape down the side of the bowl. Combine for 5 sec/reverse stir/speed 5.

4 Divide the mixture evenly between the prepared tins, then level the surface. Season the tops with salt and pepper to decorate.

5 Bake side by side, on the same shelf, for 45–50 minutes or until a skewer inserted in the centre of the loaves comes out clean and the tops are golden. Stand in the tins for 5 minutes, then transfer to a wire rack to cool completely. Serve or store.

Beef mince party pies

makes 24
preparation 45 minutes, plus chilling time,
 plus cooling time, plus 2 minutes standing time
cooking 45 minutes

1 tablespoon rosemary leaves
2 tablespoons finely chopped
 chives
1 carrot, cut into 2 cm
 (¾ inch) pieces
1 tablespoon olive oil
1 tablespoon cornflour
 (cornstarch)
2 tablespoons Vegemite or
 Marmite

2 tablespoons pizza sauce
 with garlic, onion and herbs
300 g (10½ oz) lean minced
 (ground) beef
olive oil cooking spray
3 sheets frozen shortcrust
 pastry, at room temperature
3 sheets frozen puff pastry,
 at room temperature
1 egg, whisked

The pies can be made up to
the end of step 6, then covered
in plastic wrap and frozen for
up to 3 months. Defrost in the
fridge overnight, then bake as
directed in the recipe. Cooked
pies can be stored in an airtight
container in the fridge for up to
2 days and reheated in the oven
to warm the filling and re-crisp
the pastry.

1 Add the rosemary, chives and carrot to the mixer bowl, measuring cup
   in. Chop for 5 sec/speed 7. Scrape down the side of the bowl. Chop for
   3 sec/speed 7. Scrape down the side of the bowl.

2 Add the oil to the mixer bowl, measuring cup in. Cook for 3 min/
   steaming mode/speed 1.

3 Add the cornflour, Vegemite, pizza sauce and beef to the mixer bowl,
   measuring cup in. Cook for 15 minutes/100°C/reverse stir/speed 1.
   Transfer the mixture to a heatproof bowl, cool slightly, then transfer
   to the fridge to chill.

4 Preheat the oven to 180°C (350°F)/160°C (315°F) fan-forced. Grease two
   12-hole, 1½ tablespoon capacity round-based patty pans with the oil.

5 Using a 7 cm (2¾ inch) round cutter, cut out 24 rounds from the
   shortcrust pastry and use them to line the prepared pans. Fill with the
   chilled beef mixture.

6 Using a 6 cm (2½ inch) round cutter, cut out 24 rounds from the puff
   pastry and place on top of the beef mixture, folding up the edges of the
   shortcrust pastry to overlap, and pinching together to enclose the filling.
   Brush the tops with the egg, then use a fork to prick holes in the centre
   of each pie.

7 Bake the pies in the oven, swapping the pans around on the shelves
   halfway through baking, for 20–25 minutes, or until the filling is hot and
   the pastry is cooked and golden. Stand for 2 minutes in the pans, then
   transfer the pies to a wire rack to cool further. Serve warm, at room
   temperature, or cool completely and store.

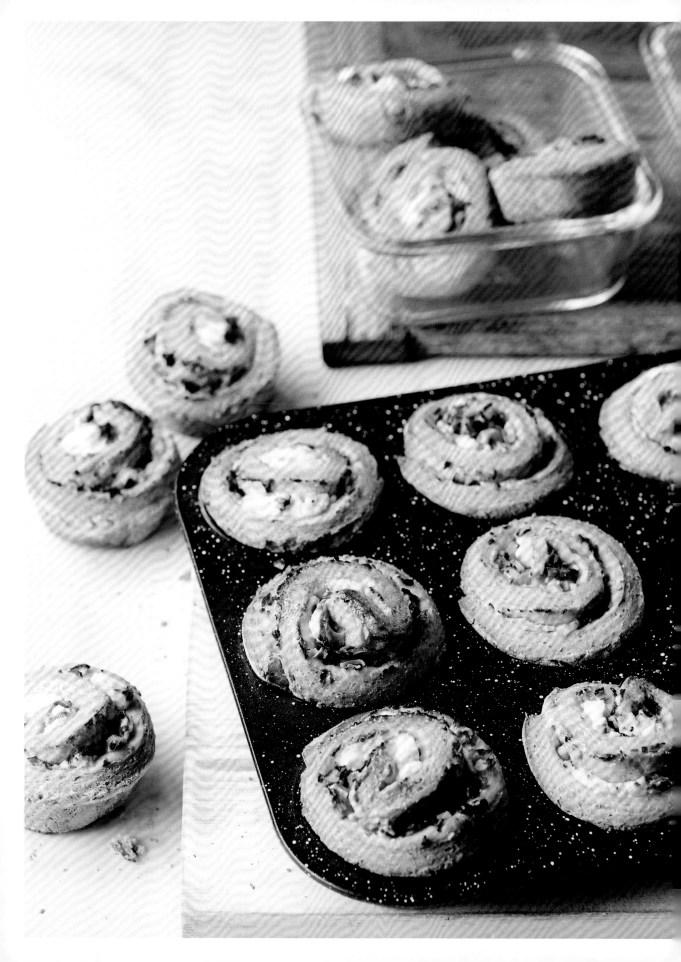

Spring onion and feta rolls

makes 18
preparation 45 minutes, plus 1½ hours proving time,
 plus 10 minutes standing time
cooking 25 minutes

250 ml (9 fl oz/1 cup) buttermilk

3 teaspoons dried instant yeast

2 teaspoons caster (superfine) sugar

50 g (1¾ oz) butter, at room temperature,
 plus extra for greasing and brushing

2 teaspoons sea salt

1 egg

225 g (8 oz/1½ cups) plain, strong bread and pizza flour,
 plus extra for dusting

450 g (1 lb/3 cups) wholemeal (whole-wheat) self-raising flour

4 spring onions (scallions), thinly sliced

200 g (7 oz) Danish feta cheese, crumbled

1 Add the buttermilk, 60 ml (2 fl oz/¼ cup) water and the yeast to the mixer bowl, measuring cup in. Heat for 3 min/50°C/speed 2. Scrape down the side of the bowl. Add the sugar, butter, salt, egg and flours to the mixer bowl, measuring cup in. Mix for 10 sec/speed 6, then knead for 2 min/kneading mode.

2 Bring the dough together with your hands, then place the dough in a lightly floured bowl, cover and stand in a warm place for 1 hour to prove or until doubled in size.

3 Preheat the oven to 200°C (400°F)/180°C (350°F) fan-forced. Liberally grease 18 holes of two 12-hole, 80 ml (2½ fl oz/⅓ cup) capacity muffin tins with the extra butter.

4 Transfer the dough to a lightly floured work surface and roll out to a 40 x 30 cm (16 x 12 inch) rectangle. Sprinkle the top evenly with the spring onion, then the feta. Using your fingertips, lightly press them into the dough. Roll up the dough tightly, from the longest side, to form a log. Cut into 18 pieces, then place each piece, cut side up, into the prepared holes of the tins. Brush the tops with the extra softened butter. Cover and stand in a warm place for 30 minutes to prove or until risen to the tops of the tins.

5 Bake the rolls for 20–25 minutes or until cooked and golden. Stand in the tins for 10 minutes, then transfer to a wire rack. Serve warm or cool completely, then store.

Asparagus and leek tarts

makes 2 tarts (serves 12)
preparation 50 minutes, plus 30 minutes chilling time,
  plus cooling time, plus 10 minutes standing time
cooking 45 minutes

500 g (1 lb 2 oz/3⅓ cups) plain
  (all-purpose) flour
400 g (14 oz) chilled butter, chopped
550 g (1 lb 4 oz/1 cup) sour cream
2 garlic cloves
2 tablespoons olive oil

2 leeks, thinly sliced
2 tablespoons lemon thyme leaves
90 g (3 oz/⅓ cup) dijon mustard
150 g (5½ oz) gouda cheese, grated
3 bunches thin asparagus, trimmed
2 eggs

1 Place the flour, butter and 250 g (9 oz/1 cup) of the sour cream in the
   mixer bowl, measuring cup in. Mix for 20 sec/speed 4. Turn out the dough
   onto a work surface lightly dusted with flour, bringing it together gently
   with your hands to form a ball. Divide in half, then flatten out each piece to
   a 4 cm (1½ inch) thick, roughly oval shape. Wrap in plastic wrap and chill
   for 30 minutes to rest. Clean the mixer bowl.

2 While the dough is chilling, add the garlic to the mixer bowl, measuring
   cup in. Chop for 5 sec/speed 4. Scrape down the side of the bowl.
   Add the oil and leek, measuring cup removed. Cook for 15 min/100°C/
   reverse stir/speed 1. Strain the mixture to remove any excess liquid, then
   transfer to a heatproof bowl. Add the lemon thyme and stir to combine,
   then set aside to cool to room temperature. Preheat the oven to 200°C
   (400°F)/180°C (350°F) fan-forced. Cut two pieces of baking paper to line
   two large baking trays. Put the paper on a work surface and place the
   trays in the oven to heat.

3 Place each piece of chilled dough onto a piece of baking paper. Using
   a rolling pin lightly dusted with flour, roll out each piece of dough to
   a rough oval, 30 cm (12 inches) in length, making sure it stays within
   the piece of paper. Brush the mustard evenly all over the pastry ovals.
   Arrange the leek mixture evenly over the bases, leaving a 5 cm (2 inch)
   border around edges. Sprinkle with half the gouda, then top with the
   asparagus. Fold up the pastry slightly at the edges, lightly pinching
   at the top. Whisk the eggs and remaining sour cream together, then
   carefully pour the mixture into the pastry shells, over the vegetables.
   Sprinkle the top with the remaining cheese.

4 Carefully slide the tarts on their paper onto the hot trays. Cook in the
   oven, swapping the trays around on the shelves halfway through baking,
   for 30 minutes or until golden. Stand on the trays for 10 minutes. Serve
   hot or transfer to a wire rack to cool completely, then store.

NOTE

Since the dough contains
a large amount of butter, it is
important that the dough is very
chilled, and the oven preheated
for at least 15 minutes before
baking, otherwise the dough
won't hold its shape.

STORAGE

The cooked tarts can be
stored in an airtight container
in the fridge for up to 3 days
or separated into portions and
placed in freezer-safe bags,
then frozen for up to 2 months.
Defrost in the fridge overnight,
then reheat in the oven to crisp.

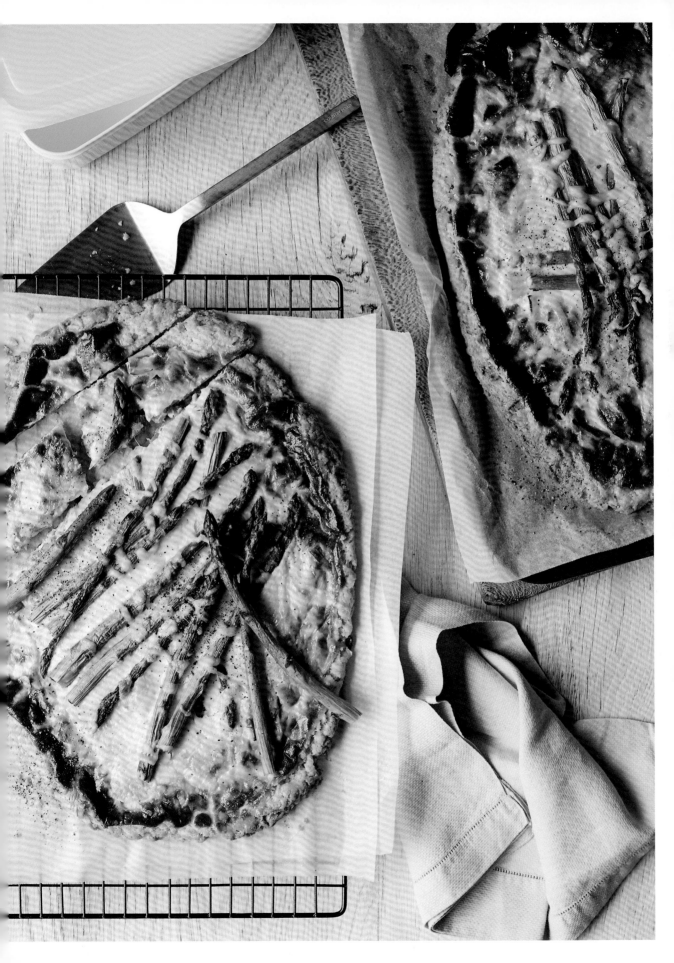

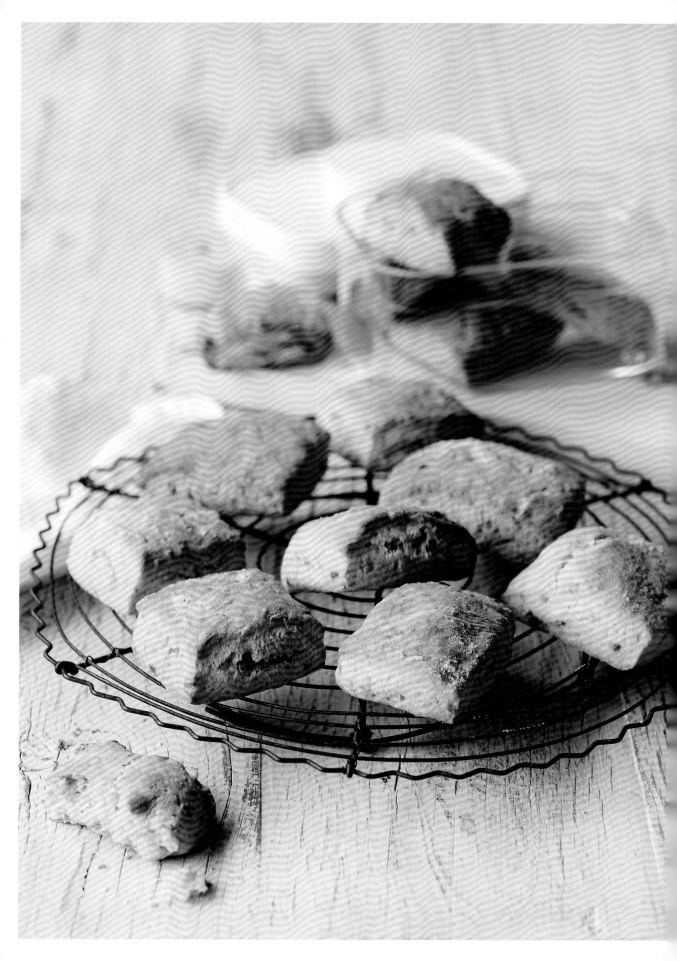

Triple cheese biscuits

makes 16
preparation 45 minutes, plus 10 minutes standing time
cooking 15 minutes

300 g (10½ oz/2 cups) plain (all-purpose) flour,
  plus extra for dusting
3 teaspoons baking powder
1 tablespoon caster (superfine) sugar
1 teaspoon sea salt
½ teaspoon sweet paprika
120 g (4¼ oz) chilled butter, chopped
30 g (1 oz/⅓ cup) grated sharp cheddar cheese
30 g (1 oz/⅓ cup) grated mild cheddar cheese
45 g (1½ oz/⅓ cup) grated mozzarella cheese
170 ml (5½ fl oz/⅔ cup) milk of choice

1 Preheat the oven to 220°C (425°F)/200°C (400°F) fan-forced. Line two
   large baking trays with baking paper.

2 Add the flour, baking powder, sugar, salt, paprika and butter to the mixer
   bowl, measuring cup in. Mix for 5 sec/speed 8 or until the mixture
   resembles breadcrumbs. Scrape down the side of the bowl.

3 Add the cheeses and milk. Mix for 20 sec/speed 5, then knead for
   20 sec/kneading mode.

4 Transfer the dough to a lightly floured work surface, bringing it together
   with your hands, then patting it out gently to a 1 cm (½ inch) thick
   square. Dip a sharp knife in the flour to dust, then cut the square into
   16 equal pieces, re-dipping the knife in the flour between each cut.
   Transfer the pieces to the prepared trays.

5 Cook the trays in the oven, swapping them around on the oven shelves
   halfway through baking, for 15 minutes or until the biscuits are cooked
   and golden. Stand on the trays for 10 minutes. Serve hot or transfer to
   a wire rack to cool completely, then store.

These are a North American
favourite and lie somewhere
between a scone and a thick
savoury cookie – full of butter
and cheese for the ultimate
moreish factor. They are great
served alongside most meals
– especially Italian fare, such
as casseroles, soups, roasts
and stews.

The cooked biscuits can be
stored in an airtight container
in a cool, dark place for up
to 3 days, in the fridge for up
to 5 days, or separated into
portions and placed in freezer-
safe bags and frozen for up to
3 months. Defrost in the fridge
overnight, then reheat in the
oven to crisp.

Iced doughnuts

makes 16 doughnuts and 16 doughnut holes
preparation 1 hour 15 minutes, plus 1–1½ hours proving time,
  plus cooling time
cooking 30 minutes

310 ml (10¾ fl oz/1¼ cups) milk
2 teaspoons instant dried yeast
50 g (1¾ oz) butter, at room
  temperature
525 g (1 lb 2¾ oz/3½ cups) plain
  (all-purpose) flour,
  plus extra for dusting
55 g (2 oz/¼ cup) caster (superfine)
  sugar
75 g (2½ oz/½ cup) currants
1 egg

hundreds and thousands
  (sprinkles), to decorate
desiccated coconut, to decorate

PINK ICING
180 g (6½ oz/1½ cups) icing
  (confectioners') sugar mixture,
  sifted
20 g (¾ oz) butter, at room
  temperature
1–2 teaspoons boiling water
2 drops red food colouring

STORAGE

The cooked, iced doughnuts
can be stored in an airtight
container in a cool, dark place
for up to 3 days or separated
into portions and placed in
freezer-safe bags, then frozen
for up to 3 months. Defrost
in the fridge overnight.

1 Add the milk, yeast and butter to the mixer bowl, measuring cup in.
   Heat for 3 min/50°C/speed 2. Scrape down the side of the bowl. Add
   the flour, sugar, currants and egg to the mixer bowl, measuring cup in.
   Knead for 2 min/kneading mode. Transfer to a lightly floured bowl, cover
   and stand for 1–1½ hours to prove or until doubled in size. Preheat the
   oven to 200°C (400°F)/180°C (350°F) fan-forced. Line three large baking
   trays with baking paper.

2 Turn the dough out onto a lightly floured surface, dust the top with
   a little more flour, then roll out to a 1 cm (½ inch) thickness. Use an
   8 cm (3¼ inch) round cutter to cut out rounds from the dough, as close
   together as possible, and re-roll the offcuts to cut out more rounds until
   you have 16. Use a 3 cm (1¼ inch) round cutter to cut out smaller
   rounds from the centre of each (the 'holes'). Transfer the doughnuts
   and doughnut holes to the prepared trays.

3 Cook in the oven, swapping the trays around on the shelves halfway
   through baking, for 12–15 minutes or until cooked and light golden.
   Stand on the trays for 5 minutes, then transfer to a wire rack to cool
   completely.

4 Make the pink icing by adding all the ingredients to the mixer bowl,
   measuring cup in. Mix for 10 sec/speed 4. Scrape down the side of
   the bowl. Mix for 5 sec/speed 4 or until smooth. Spread the pink icing
   evenly over the cooled doughnuts and doughnut holes and immediately
   dip the doughnuts into the hundreds and thousands, and the doughnut
   holes into the desiccated coconut. Leave to set, then serve or store.

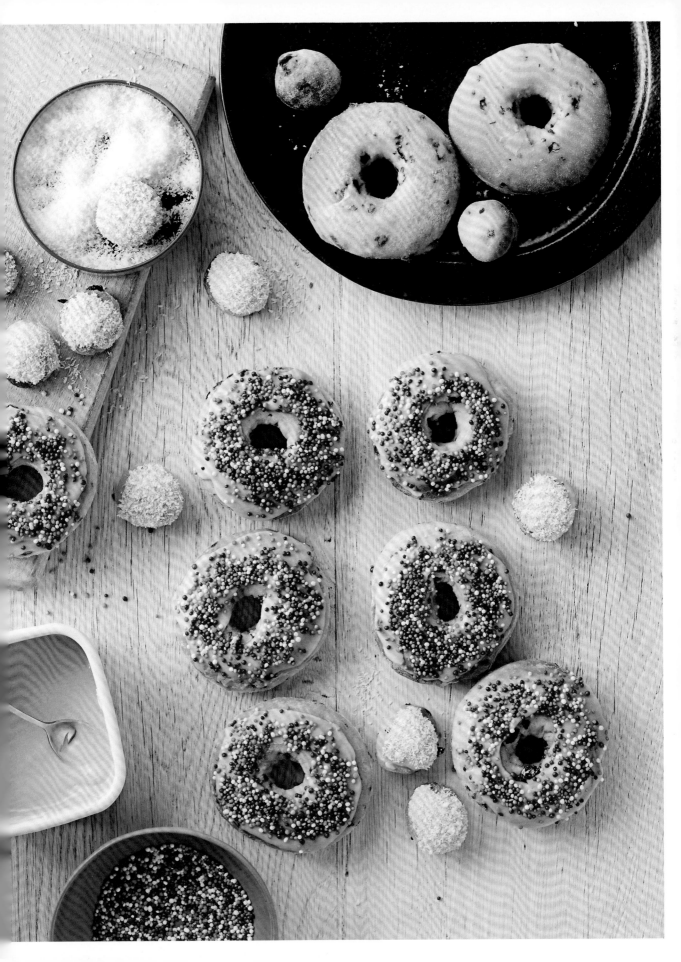

Tropical cake

serves 24
preparation 45 minutes, plus cooling time
cooking 45 minutes

6 medium ripe bananas, cut into 3
250 ml (9 fl oz/1 cup) macadamia oil
4 eggs
370 g (13 oz/2 cups) brown sugar
3 teaspoons ground cinnamon
225 g (8 oz/1½ cups) plain (all-purpose) flour
225 g (8 oz/1½ cups) self-raising flour
3 teaspoons baking powder
90 g (3 oz/1 cup) desiccated coconut
500 g (1 lb 2 oz) tinned crushed pineapple in syrup, drained,
  reserving 170 ml (5½ fl oz/⅔ cup) of the syrup from the tins
155 g (5½ oz/1 cup) macadamia nuts, roasted and finely chopped

CREAM CHEESE FROSTING
250 g (9 oz) cream cheese, at room temperature
1 tablespoon finely grated lime zest (see note)
360 g (12¾ oz/3 cups) icing (confectioners') sugar mixture, sifted

1 Preheat the oven to 180°C (350°F)/160°C (315°F) fan-forced. Line the
   base and sides of a 37.5 x 25 x 3 cm (14¾ x 10 x 1¼ inch) non-stick
   baking tray with baking paper.

2 Add the bananas to the mixer bowl, measuring cup in. Mash for 5 sec/
   speed 6. Scrape down the side of the bowl.

3 Add the oil, eggs, sugar, cinnamon, flours and baking powder to the
   mixer bowl, measuring cup in. Mix for 5 sec/speed 5. Scrape down
   the side of the bowl.

4 Add the coconut, pineapple and syrup to the mixer bowl, measuring
   cup in. Mix for 10 sec/reverse stir/speed 5. Transfer the mixture to the
   prepared tray and level the surface. Clean the mixer bowl.

5 Bake the cake for 40–45 minutes or until a skewer inserted in the centre
   comes out clean and the cake is golden. Cool completely in the tray.

6 Make the cream cheese frosting by adding the cream cheese, lime zest
   and icing sugar to the mixer bowl, measuring cup in. Mix for 20 sec/
   speed 5.

7 Spread the cream cheese frosting evenly over the cake. Sprinkle with
   the macadamia nuts, then slice and serve or store.

NOTE

You'll need 4 large limes for the
zest. Store the left-over zested
limes in an airtight container
in the fridge for up to 1 week,
or juice and freeze the excess
juice in ice cube trays for up
to 2 months.

STORAGE

The cooked, frosted cake
can be stored in an airtight
container in the fridge for
up to 3 days, or chilled, then
separated into portions, placed
in freezer-safe bags and frozen
for up to 2 months. Defrost in
the fridge overnight.

Cinnamon apple teacakes

makes 24
preparation 45 minutes, plus cooling time
cooking 20 minutes

3 green apples, peeled, cored and quartered
250 g (9 oz) butter, at room temperature
220 g (7¾ oz/1 cup) caster (superfine) sugar
3 teaspoons pure vanilla extract
4 eggs
250 g (9 oz/1⅔ cups) self-raising flour
2 teaspoons baking powder
1½ teaspoons ground cinnamon
icing (confectioners') sugar, to dust

1   Preheat the oven to 180°C (350°F)/160°C (315°F) fan-forced. Line two 12-hole, 80 ml (2½ fl oz/⅓ cup) capacity muffin tins with paper cases.

2   Cut each apple quarter in half crossways and set aside.

3   Add the butter, caster sugar, vanilla, eggs, flour, baking powder and cinnamon to the mixer bowl, measuring cup in. Mix for 20 sec/speed 6. Divide the mixture evenly among the holes in the prepared tins.

4   Working one at a time, take a piece of apple, slice it thinly lengthways, then arrange it in the centre of the mixture in a muffin hole.

5   Bake for 18–20 minutes, swapping the tins around on the oven shelves halfway through baking, until a skewer inserted in the centre of a teacake comes out clean and golden. Stand in the tins for 3 minutes, then transfer to a wire rack to cool completely. Serve dusted with icing sugar or store.

STORAGE

The cooked cakes can be stored in an airtight container in a cool, dark place for up to 3 days, in the fridge for up to 5 days or separated into portions and placed in freezer-safe bags and frozen for up to 2 months. Defrost in the fridge overnight.

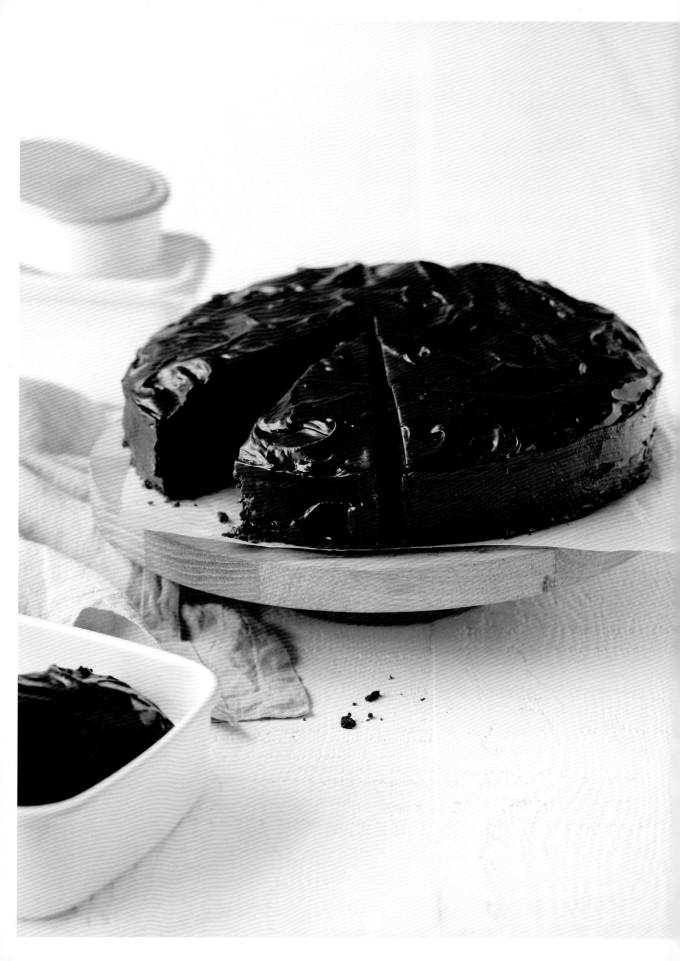

Rich mocha mud cake

serves 12
preparation 45 minutes, plus 30 minutes standing time,
  plus cooling time
cooking 1 hour 20 minutes

200 g (7 oz) 70% dark chocolate, broken into pieces
250 g (9 oz) butter, chopped
250 ml (9 fl oz/1 cup) strong-brewed plunger coffee
60 ml (2 fl oz/¼ cup) coffee-flavoured liqueur
440 g (15½ oz/2 cups) caster (superfine) sugar
225 g (8 oz/1½ cups) plain (all-purpose) flour
2 teaspoons baking powder
50 g (1¾ oz/½ cup) almond meal
4 eggs

GANACHE
250 g (9 oz) milk cooking chocolate
250 g (9 oz) dark cooking chocolate
170 ml (5½ fl oz/⅔ cup) thin (pouring/whipping) cream

STORAGE

The cooked, ganache-covered
cake can be stored in an
airtight container in a cool,
dark place for up to 2 days,
in the fridge for up to 5 days,
or separated into portions and
placed in freezer-safe bags,
then frozen for up to 3 months.
Defrost in the fridge overnight,
then bring to room temperature
before serving.

1 Preheat the oven to 160°C (315°F)/140°C (275°F) fan-forced. Line the
   base and side of a 22 cm (8½ inch) round spring-form cake tin with
   baking paper.

2 Add the dark chocolate to the mixer bowl, measuring cup in. Grate for
   8 sec/speed 7. Scrape down the side of the bowl. Add the butter, coffee
   and coffee liqueur to the mixer bowl, measuring cup in. Cook for 2 min/
   50°C/speed 2 or until melted and smooth.

3 Add the sugar, flour, baking powder, almond meal and eggs to the mixer
   bowl, measuring cup in. Mix for 20 sec/speed 5 or until combined – the
   mixture will be runny. Pour the mixture into the prepared tin and level
   the surface. Clean the mixer bowl.

4 Bake the cake for 1 hour 15 minutes or until a skewer inserted in the
   centre comes out clean. Stand in the tin for 30 minutes, then transfer
   to a wire rack to cool completely.

5 Meanwhile, make the ganache by adding the chocolates to the mixer
   bowl, measuring cup in. Grate for 8 sec/speed 7. Scrape down the
   side of the bowl. Add the cream to the mixer bowl, measuring cup in.
   Cook for 2 min/50°C/speed 2, or until melted. Transfer the mixture to
   a heatproof bowl. Stand at room temperature, stirring occasionally, until
   completely cooled and thickened (to a spreadable consistency).

6 Spread the ganache evenly over the cake, then slice and serve or store.

Salted caramel slice

makes 24 pieces
preparation 30 minutes, plus cooling time,
   plus 2 hours chilling time
cooking 45 minutes

250 g (9 oz) butter, chopped
300 g (10½ oz/2 cups) wholemeal (whole-wheat)
   self-raising flour
180 g (6½ oz/2 cups) desiccated coconut
220 g (7¾ oz/1 cup) white sugar
100 g (3½ oz) pitted medjool dates
1.2 kg (2 lb 12 oz) tinned condensed milk
135 g (4¾ oz/½ cup) hulled tahini
200 g (7 oz) dark chocolate baking chips
pink sea salt flakes, to sprinkle

STORAGE

The cooked slice can be stored
in an airtight container in the
fridge for up to 1 week, or
separated into portions and
individually wrapped in plastic
wrap, then foil, and placed in
a freezer-safe container and
frozen for up to 2 months.
Defrost in the fridge overnight.

1 Preheat the oven to 180°C (350°F)/160°C (315°F) fan-forced. Line the
   base and sides of a 37.5 x 25 x 3 cm (14¾ x 10 x 1¼ inch) non-stick
   baking tray with baking paper.

2 Add the butter to the mixer bowl, measuring cup in. Cook for 2 min/
   50°C/speed 1 or until melted. Scrape down the side of the bowl.

3 Add the flour, coconut and sugar to the mixer bowl, measuring cup in.
   Mix for 10 sec/speed 4. Scrape down the side of the bowl. Mix for
   10 sec/speed 4. Transfer the mixture to the prepared tray, pressing
   down firmly to evenly cover the base. Bake for 10 minutes or until
   cooked and very light golden. Cool completely in the tray. Clean the
   mixer bowl.

4 Add the dates to the mixer bowl, measuring cup in. Chop for 5 sec/
   speed 7. Scrape down the side of the bowl.

5 Add the condensed milk to the mixer bowl, measuring cup removed
   and the steamer basket set over the lid. Cook for 20 min/100°C/speed 3.
   Cool for 2 minutes.

6 Add the tahini to the mixer bowl, measuring cup removed. Mix for
   10 sec/speed 3. Pour the mixture over the base in the prepared tray,
   levelling the surface. Sprinkle evenly with the chocolate chips.

7 Bake for 10 minutes, then remove from the oven and sprinkle the top
   with sea salt. Cool completely in the tray, then chill for 2 hours or until
   set. Slice and serve or store.

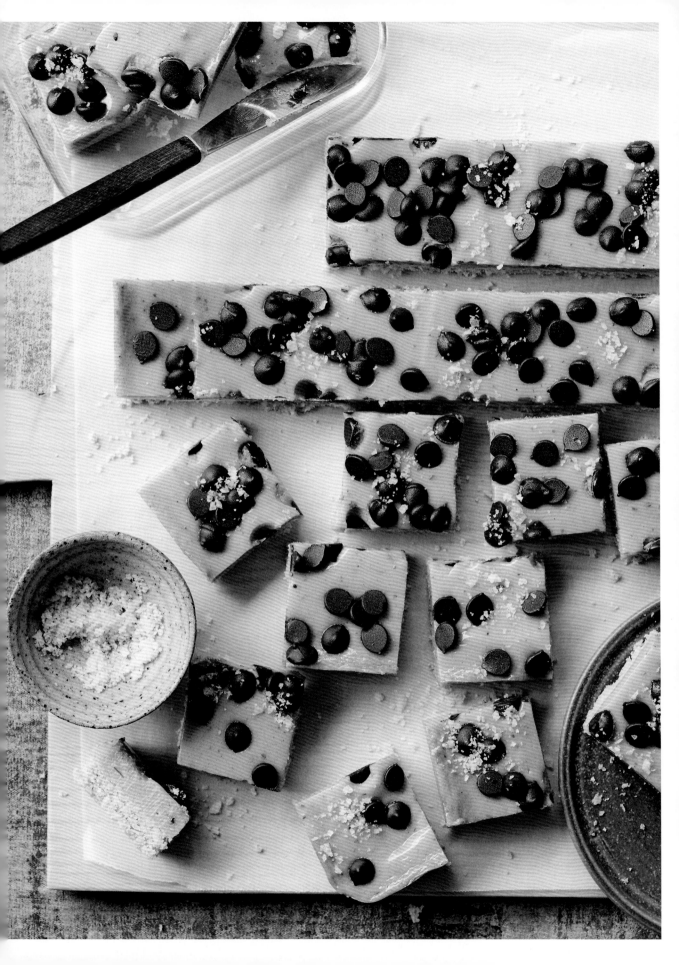

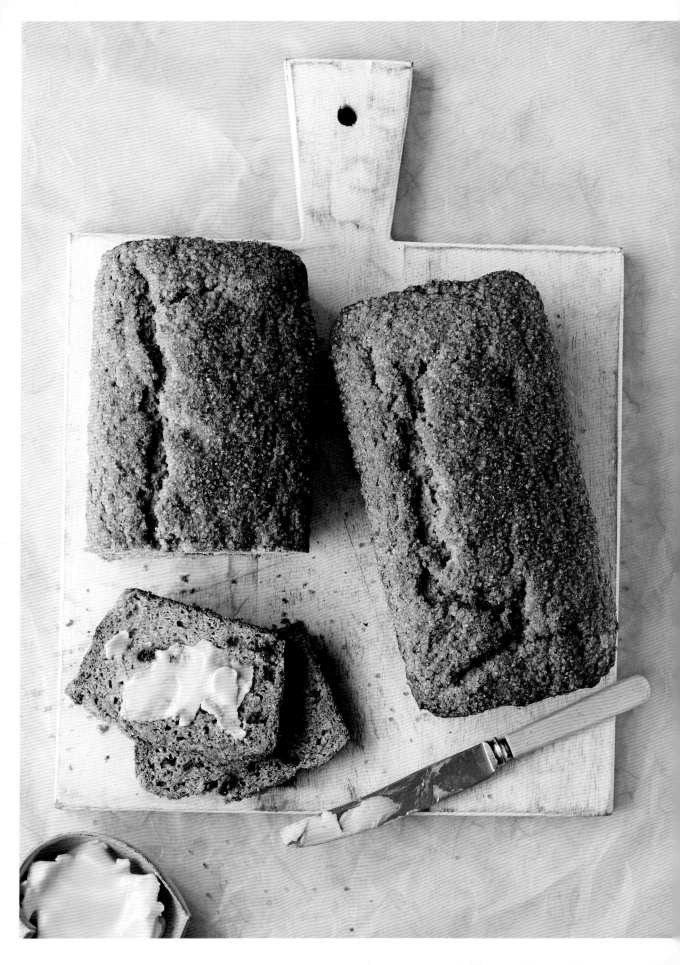

Date and banana loaf

makes 2 loaves (serves 16)
preparation 20 minutes, plus 30 minutes standing time
cooking 55 minutes

6 medium ripe bananas, cut into 3
100 g (3½ oz) butter
125 ml (4 fl oz/½ cup) pure maple syrup
500 g (1 lb 2 oz) store-bought unsweetened apple purée
1 teaspoon ground cinnamon
80 g (2¾ oz/½ cup) chopped pitted dried dates
600 g (1 lb 5 oz/4 cups) wholemeal (whole-wheat)
  self-raising flour
3 teaspoons baking powder
50 g (1¾ oz/¼ cup) raw (demerara) sugar

STORAGE

The cooked loaves can be stored in an airtight container in the fridge for up to 5 days, or separated into portions and placed in freezer-safe bags and frozen for up to 3 months. Defrost in the fridge overnight and toast before serving.

1 Preheat the oven to 180°C (350°F)/160°C (315°F) fan-forced. Line the base and sides of two 22 x 10 x 7 cm (8½ x 4 x 2¾ inch) loaf (bar) tins with baking paper.

2 Add the bananas to the mixer bowl, measuring cup in. Mash for 5 sec/speed 6. Scrape down the side of the bowl.

3 Add the butter, maple syrup and apple purée to the mixer bowl, measuring cup in. Mix for 20 sec/speed 4. Scrape down the side of the bowl.

4 Add the cinnamon, dates, flour and baking powder to the mixer bowl, measuring cup in. Mix for 20 sec/speed 4 – the mixture will just be combined, do not overmix. Scrape down the side of the bowl. Divide the mixture evenly among the prepared tins and level the surface. Sprinkle the tops evenly with the raw sugar.

5 Bake the loaves side by side in the oven for 50–55 minutes or until a skewer inserted in the centre comes out clean and they are golden. Stand in the tins for 30 minutes, then transfer to a wire rack. Serve warm, or cool completely and store.

Made-to-order vanilla cookies

makes 30 cookies
preparation 40 minutes, plus 30 minutes freezing time, plus cooling time
cooking 45 minutes

250 g (9 oz) butter, at room temperature
165 g (5¾ oz/¾ cup) caster (superfine) sugar
3 teaspoons vanilla bean paste
1 egg
375 g (13 oz/2½ cups) plain soft, pastry/cake flour, plus extra for dusting

1   Add the butter and sugar to the mixer bowl, measuring cup in. Mix for 30 sec/speed 4. Scrape down the side of the bowl. Mix for 30 sec/speed 4. Scrape down the side of the bowl.

2   Add the vanilla and egg to the mixer bowl, measuring cup in. Mix for 1 min/speed 4. Scrape down the side of the bowl.

3   Add the flour to the mixer bowl, measuring cup in. Mix for 15 sec/speed 4. Scrape down the side of the bowl. Mix for 15 sec/speed 4. Transfer the mixture to a lightly floured surface and bring together in a ball. Divide into two equal portions, then shape each portion into a smooth 15 cm (6 inch) long log. Wrap each log in plastic wrap. Freeze for 30 minutes or until almost firm.

4   Preheat the oven to 180°C (350°F)/160°C (315°F) fan-forced. Line three large baking trays with baking paper.

5   Using a sharp knife, slice the logs into 1 cm (½ inch) wide rounds. Transfer the rounds to the prepared trays. Bake each tray of cookies for 12–15 minutes or until they are cooked, light golden and crisp. Stand on the trays for 5 minutes. Serve warm or transfer to a wire rack to cool completely, then store.

NOTE

This is the best cookie dough to have on hand in the freezer at all times. It's perfect to slice and bake as you need and great for when someone pops over, or you just want to treat yourself! You can either add 40 g (1½ oz/⅓ cup) hundreds and thousands (sprinkles), 1 tablespoon finely grated lemon or orange zest, or 1 teaspoon ground cinnamon to the dough mixture when you add the flour for mixing.

STORAGE

The cooked cookies can be stored in an airtight container in a cool, dark place for up to 5 days, or the uncooked frozen logs of dough can be stored for up to 2 months. Stand at room temperature for 5 minutes, slice what you need and bake, then re-wrap and freeze.

Festive panforte

makes 2 (serves 24)
preparation 40 minutes, plus cooling time
cooking 40 minutes

200 g (7 oz) dry-roasted almonds, chopped
200 g (7 oz) dry-roasted hazelnuts, skins removed
220 g (7¾ oz/1½ cups) sweetened dried cranberries
170 g (6 oz/1 cup) raisins
185 g (6½ oz/1 cup) chopped soft and juicy dried figs
1 tablespoon ground cinnamon
1 tablespoon ground ginger
2 teaspoons mixed spice
200 g (7 oz/1⅓ cups) plain (all-purpose) flour
40 g (1½ oz/⅓ cup) unsweetened cocoa powder,
  plus extra for dusting
200 g (7 oz) 70% dark chocolate, broken into pieces
110 g (3¾ oz/2 cups) caster (superfine) sugar
250 ml (9 fl oz/1 cup) honey

1 Preheat the oven to 150°C (300°F)/130°C (250°F) fan-forced. Line the base and sides of two 20 cm (8 inch) round spring-form cake tins with baking paper.

2 Add the almonds, hazelnuts, cranberries, raisins, figs, spices, flour and cocoa to a very large heatproof bowl. Stir to combine, making sure that all the nuts and fruit are evenly coated in the flour and cocoa powder. Set aside.

3 Add the dark chocolate to the mixer bowl, measuring cup in. Grate for 8 sec/speed 7. Scrape down the side of the bowl. Melt for 3 min/ 50°C/speed 1. Scrape down the side of the bowl. Cook for 2 min/50°C/ speed 1 or until melted and smooth. Transfer to a heatproof bowl, cover with a tea towel (dish towel) to keep warm. Set aside. No need to clean the bowl.

4 Add the sugar and honey to the mixer bowl, measuring cup in. Cook for 5 min/steaming mode/speed 1. Pour the mixture over the nut mixture in the bowl, adding the melted chocolate at the same time. Working quickly, stir together until well combined. Divide evenly among the prepared tins, pressing down firmly to cover the bases of the tins evenly.

5 Bake the panforte side by side in the oven for 25–30 minutes or until the edges are just firm and the centres still slightly soft (the panforte will set on cooling). Cool completely in the tins. Remove and dust with the extra cocoa, then slice and serve or store.

NOTE

This makes a delicious baked treat at holiday time and is ideal as a baked gift at any time of year. It's delicious served with a strong coffee or your favourite evening tipple.

STORAGE

Cooked panforte can be wrapped in plastic wrap and stored in an airtight container in a cool, dark place for up to 2 months. If gifting panforte, you can wrap either whole panforte, or slices, in baking paper, tied together with kitchen twine.

lunchbox fillers

These lunchbox fillers are all freezer-friendly and great for using up those end-of-week fridge and pantry 'bits', as well as the pieces of fruit that seem to boomerang back home in kids' lunchboxes. These delicious recipes are lower in sugar than the store-bought versions, but are high in energy and brain-boosting foods for children. They're also great for adults to take to work, or make wonderful snacks to have handy in the freezer to thaw out when you feel like them. Next time you're out and about all day with the kids, take some of these along to banish those 'hangry' episodes. Storage tips are provided for all recipes.

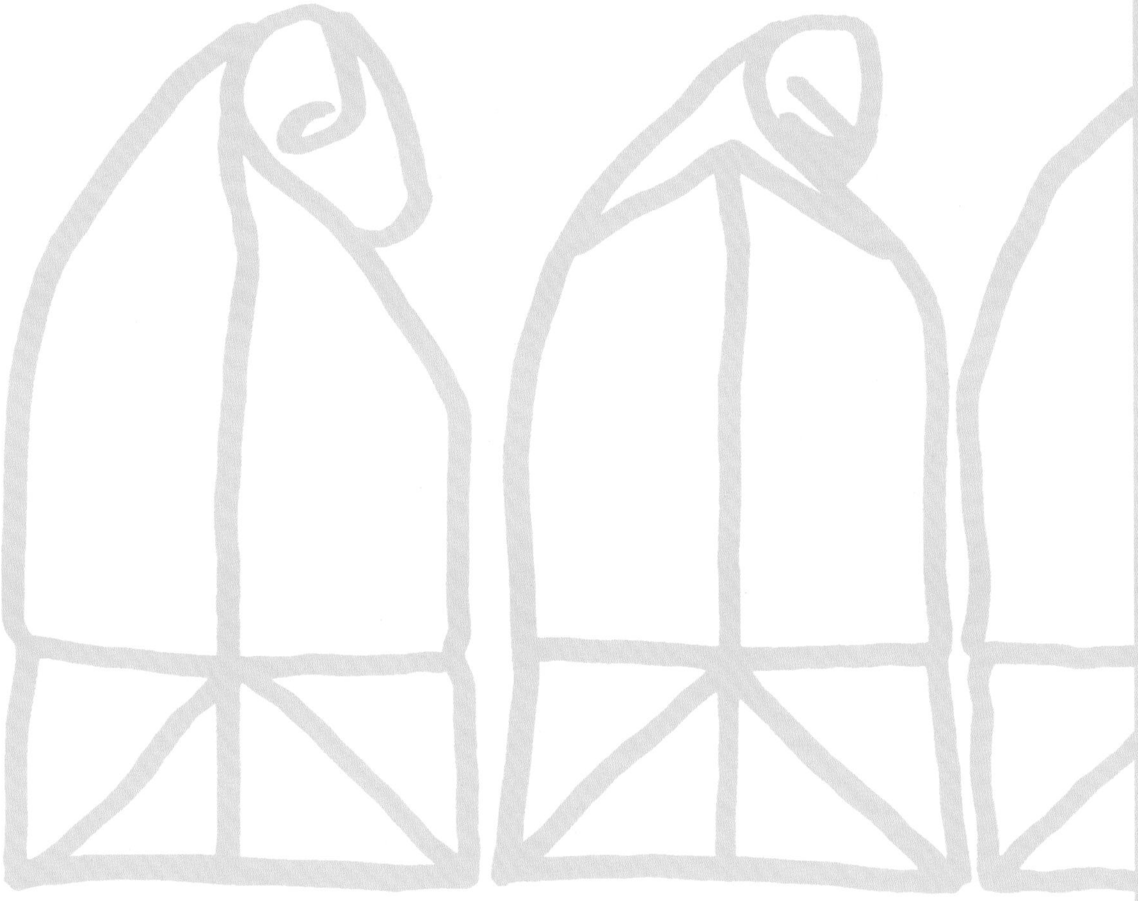

Ham and hidden vegie tomato scrolls

makes 50
preparation 1 hour, plus 2 hours chilling time,
  plus cooling time
cooking 50 minutes

2 celery stalks, cut into 2 cm (¾ inch) pieces
2 carrots, cut into 2 cm (¾ inch) pieces
150 g (5½ oz) cauliflower florets
2 tablespoons chopped chives
240 g (8¾ oz/2 cups) grated three-cheese mix
  (mozzarella, cheddar, parmesan)
300 g (10½ oz) shredded ham
125 ml (4 fl oz/½ cup) reduced-sugar
  tomato sauce (ketchup)
5 sheets frozen puff pastry, at room temperature
2 eggs, whisked

1 Add the celery, carrot, cauliflower and chives to the mixer bowl, measuring cup in. Chop for 5 sec/speed 5, or until finely chopped. Scrape down the side of the bowl.

2 Add the cheese and ham to the mixer bowl, measuring cup in. Chop for 5 sec/speed 5, or until finely chopped. Scrape down the side of the bowl.

3 Add the tomato sauce to the mixer bowl, measuring cup in. Combine for 3 sec/speed 7, or until just combined.

4 Spread the mixture evenly among the pastry sheets, leaving a 2 cm (¾ inch) border on one side. Brush the edges of the pastry with egg, then roll up to form a log and to enclose the filling. Wrap each roll in plastic wrap and chill for 2 hours (see storage note). Chill the remaining whisked egg.

5 Preheat the oven to 200°C (400°F)/180°C (350°F) fan-forced. Line four large baking trays with baking paper.

6 Brush the rolls with the remaining whisked egg. Cut each roll into 10 slices, then place, cut side up, on the prepared trays. Bake two trays of scrolls at a time, swapping the trays around in the oven halfway through baking, for 20–25 minutes or until cooked, puffed and golden. Cool the scrolls completely on the trays.

STORAGE

After wrapping the scrolls in plastic wrap, you can choose to freeze, then defrost, cut and bake at a later date. Frozen uncooked rolls will keep for up to 3 months. Defrost in the fridge overnight before cutting. The scrolls will keep in an airtight container in the fridge for up to 5 days. Separate into smaller portions in freezer-safe bags and freeze for up to 3 months.

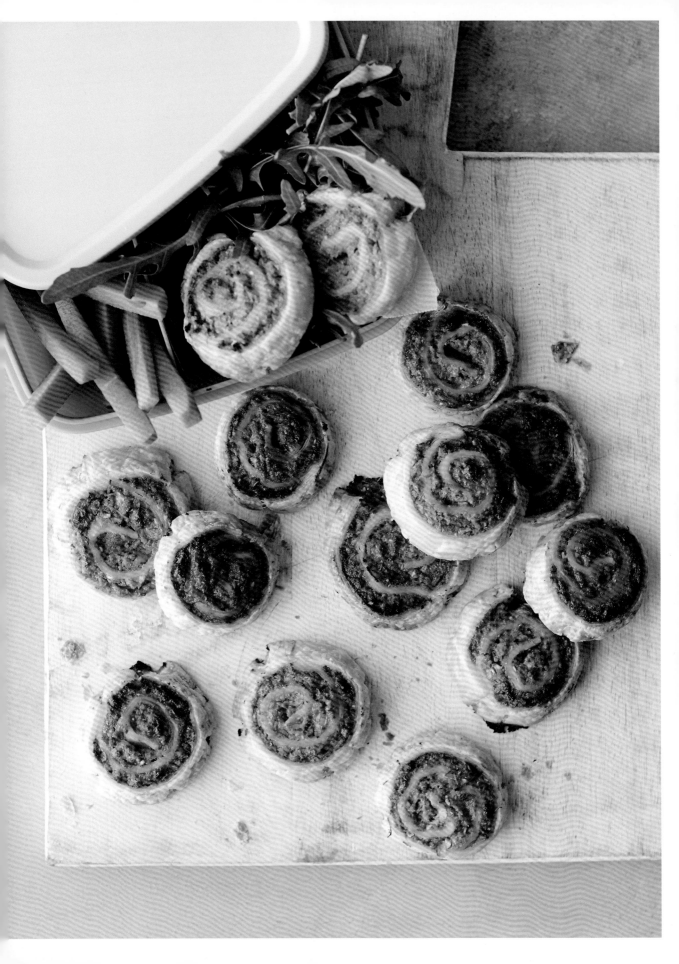

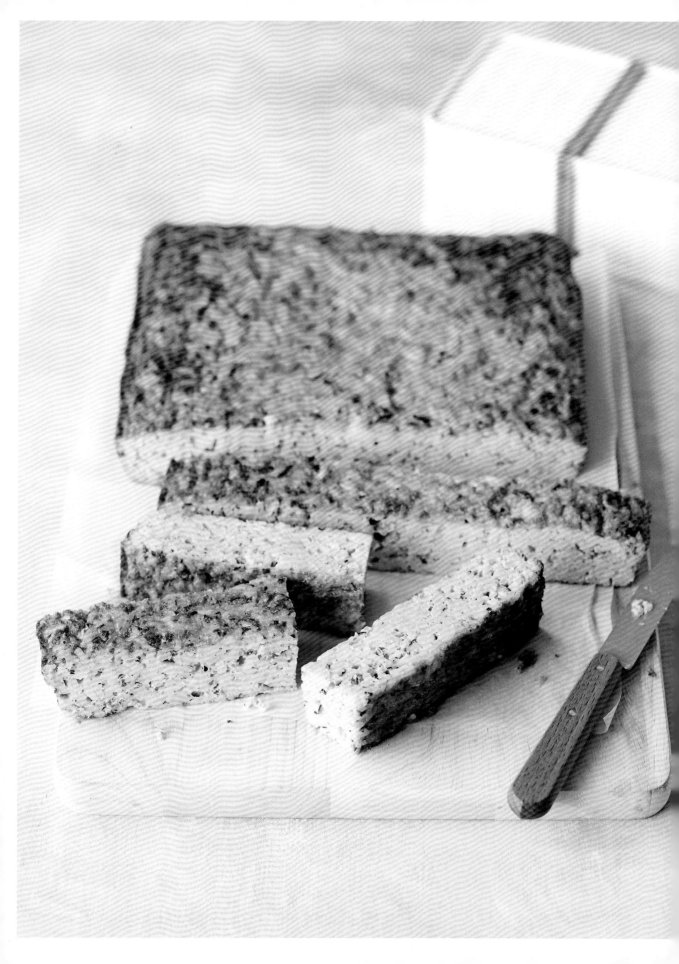

Zucchini and rice slice

makes 24 pieces
preparation 30 minutes, plus cooling time
cooking 35 minutes

4 zucchini (courgettes),
  cut into 2 cm (¾ inch) pieces
1 small bunch chives,
  cut into 2 cm (¾ inch) pieces
200 g (7 oz/2 cups) grated mild
  cheddar cheese
12 eggs
600 g (1 lb 5 oz/4 cups) cooked white rice

STORAGE

The slice will keep in an airtight container in the fridge for up to 5 days. Separate into smaller portions in freezer-safe bags and freeze for up to 3 months.

1   Preheat the oven to 180°C (350°F)/160°C (315°F) fan-forced. Line the base and sides of a 35 cm x 25 x 2 cm (14 x 10 x ¾ inch) baking tray with baking paper.

2   Add the zucchini and chives to the mixer bowl, measuring cup in. Chop for 3 sec/speed 7, or until finely chopped. Scrape down the side of the bowl.

3   Add the cheese and eggs to the mixer bowl, measuring cup in. Mix for 5 sec/speed 4. Scrape down the side of the bowl.

4   Add the rice to the mixer bowl, measuring cup in. Stir for 5 sec/ reverse stir/speed 4 until well combined.

5   Pour the mixture into the prepared tray. Bake the slice for 30–35 minutes or until cooked and golden. Cool completely in the tray. Remove and cut into pieces.

Sausage and tomato bread quiches

makes 24
preparation 45 minutes, plus cooling time
cooking 35 minutes

4 thin chicken, beef, pork or vegetarian sausages
olive oil cooking spray
24 slices sandwich bread, crusts removed
200 g (7 oz) sweet baby tomatoes,
  sliced into rounds
8 eggs
125 ml (4 fl oz/½ cup) thickened (whipping) cream
½ teaspoon dried mixed herbs

1 Place a non-stick frying pan over medium heat. Cook the sausages,
   turning occasionally, for 8–10 minutes or until cooked and golden.
   Transfer to a board and allow to cool slightly. Thinly slice the sausages
   into rounds.

2 Preheat the oven to 200°C (400°F)/180°C (350°F) fan-forced. Spray
   two 12-hole, 80 ml (2½ fl oz/⅓ cup) capacity muffin tins with the oil
   to grease.

3 Using a rolling pin, roll out each slice of bread until thin. Spray both
   sides of the bread with the oil, then carefully push the slices into the
   holes in the prepared muffin tins to line. Fill evenly with the sausage
   and tomato mixture.

4 Add the eggs, cream and mixed herbs to the mixer bowl, measuring
   cup in. Mix for 30 sec/speed 4.

5 Pour the egg mixture evenly over the filling in the bread cases in the
   tins. Bake the quiches for 15–20 minutes, swapping the trays around
   in the oven halfway through baking, or until cooked and golden. Cool in
   the tins for 3 minutes, then transfer to a wire rack to cool completely.

NOTE

Every time you have some stale
left-over bread slices at the
end of the week, pop them in
freezer-safe bags, then into the
freezer. Once you've collected
enough pieces, simply defrost
in the fridge, then use them for
this recipe.

STORAGE

The quiches will keep in an
airtight container in the fridge
for up to 3 days. Separate into
smaller portions in freezer-safe
bags and freeze for up to
2 months.

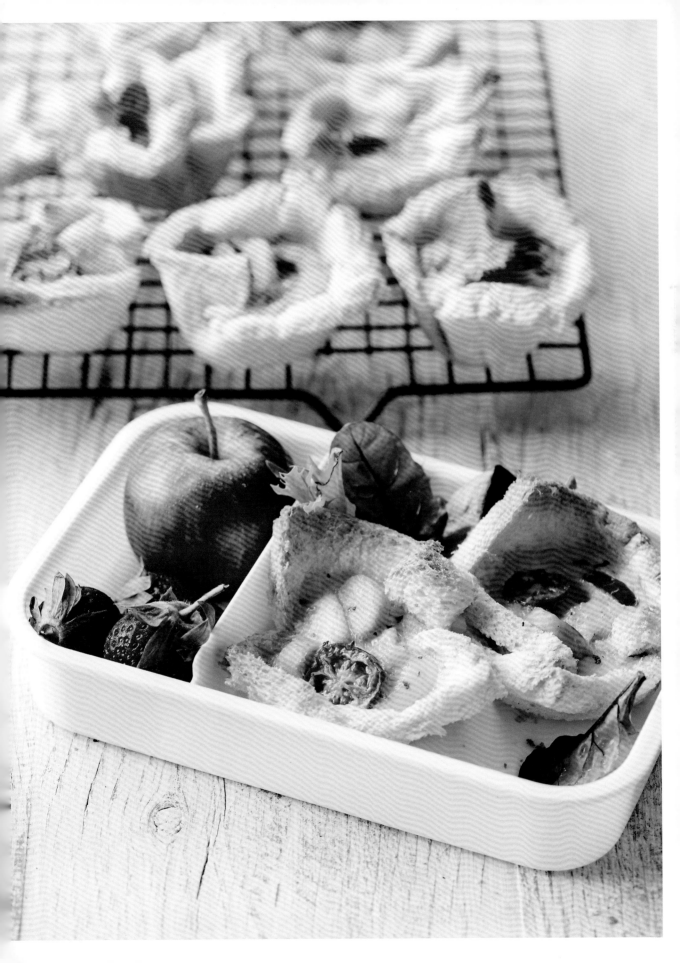

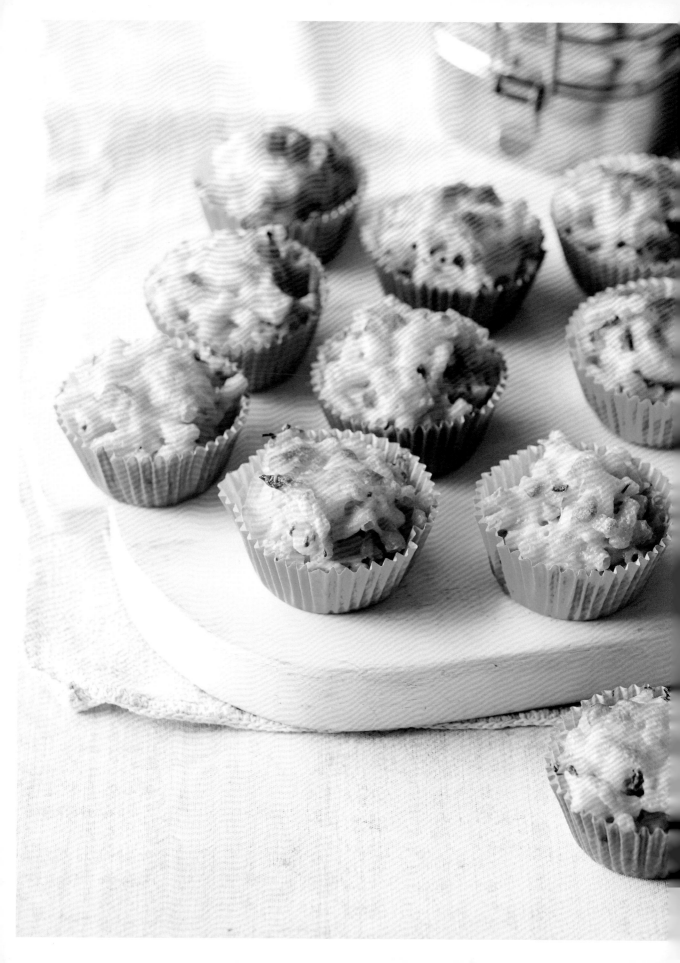

Baked chicken macaroni cheese

makes 24
preparation 30 minutes, plus cooling time
cooking 45 minutes

280 g (10 oz/2 cups) small dried macaroni
300 g (10½ oz) barbecued chicken meat, chopped
2 tablespoons finely chopped chives
30 g (1 oz) butter
2 tablespoons plain (all-purpose) flour
250 ml (9 fl oz/1 cup) milk of choice
120 g (4¼ oz/1 cup) grated three-cheese mix (mozzarella,
   cheddar and parmesan), plus 60 g (2¼ oz/½ cup) extra for topping

STORAGE

The macaroni cheese will
keep in an airtight container
in the fridge for up to 3 days.
Separate into smaller portions
in freezer-safe bags and freeze
for up to 2 months.

1 Preheat the oven to 180°C (350°F)/160°C (315°F) fan-forced.
   Double-line two 12-hole, 80 ml (2½ fl oz/⅓ cup) capacity muffin
   tins with paper cases.

2 Cook the macaroni according to the packet directions, but minus
   2 minutes' cooking time (they will continue cooking when baked).
   Drain well. Transfer to a large heatproof bowl. Add the chicken and
   chives. Mix to combine.

3 Add the butter, flour and milk to the mixer bowl, measuring cup in.
   Cook for 6 min/90°C/speed 4.

4 Add the cheese to the mixer bowl, measuring cup in. Cook for
   2 min/90°C/speed 2. Pour over the macaroni mixture in the bowl.
   Mix to combine.

5 Divide the mixture evenly among the holes in the prepared tins, then
   sprinkle the tops with the extra cheese. Bake for 20–25 minutes or until
   golden. Cool in the tins for 5 minutes, then transfer to a wire rack to
   cool completely.

Corn and feta muffins

makes 48
preparation 30 minutes, plus cooling time
cooking 20 minutes

375 g (13 oz/2½ cups) wholemeal (whole-wheat)
  self-raising flour
185 ml (6 fl oz/¾ cup) milk of choice
1 egg
125 ml (4 fl oz/½ cup) macadamia oil
125 g (4½ oz) tinned creamed corn
100 g (3½ oz) Danish feta cheese, crumbled

STORAGE

The muffins will keep in an airtight container in the fridge for up to 5 days. Separate into smaller portions in freezer-safe bags and freeze for up to 1 month.

1 Preheat the oven to 180°C (350°F)/160°C (315°F) fan-forced. Line two 24-hole, 2 tablespoon capacity mini muffin tins with paper cases.

2 Add the flour, milk, egg, oil and corn to the mixer bowl, measuring cup in. Mix for 5 sec/speed 4. Scrape down the side of the bowl.

3 Add the feta to the mixer bowl, measuring cup in. Mix for 20 sec/reverse stir/speed 1.

4 Spoon the mixture evenly among the holes in the prepared tins. Bake the muffins for 15–20 minutes or until a skewer inserted in the centre comes out clean and the tops are golden. Cool in the tins for 5 minutes, then transfer to a wire rack to cool completely.

Bolognese meatballs

makes 30
preparation 40 minutes, plus cooling time
cooking 45 minutes

700 g (1 lb 9 oz) lean beef topside, all visible
  fat removed, cut into 2 cm (¾ inch) pieces
2 celery stalks, cut into 2 cm (¾ inch) pieces
1 carrot, cut into 2 cm (¾ inch) pieces
30 g (1 oz/¼ cup) shaved parmesan cheese
2 slices day-old sandwich bread, torn into 2 cm
  (¾ inch) pieces
60 ml (2 fl oz/¼ cup) pizza sauce
1 egg
olive oil cooking spray

The meatballs will keep in an
airtight container in the fridge
for up to 3 days. Separate into
smaller portions in freezer-
safe bags and freeze for up
to 3 months.

1 Add the beef to the mixer bowl, measuring cup in. Mince (grind) for
   10 sec/speed 7. Scrape down the side of the bowl. Mince for 15 sec/
   speed 7 or until fine. Transfer to a large bowl.

2 Add the celery and carrot to the mixer bowl, measuring cup in.
   Chop for 10 sec/speed 7. Scrape down the side of the bowl.

3 Add the parmesan, bread, pizza sauce and egg, measuring cup in.
   Blend for 10 sec/speed 9.

4 Transfer the vegetable mixture to the beef in the bowl. Mix until well
   combined. Roll 1 tablespoon measures of the mixture into balls.

5 Place a large non-stick frying pan over medium–high heat. Spray
   with oil. Cook the meatballs in batches, turning occasionally, for
   12–15 minutes or until cooked and golden. Transfer to a plate
   to cool completely.

Toasted muesli and sesame balls

makes 45
preparation 45 minutes, plus chilling time
cooking 1 minute

400 g (14 oz/2 cups) pitted prunes
100 g (3½ oz) unsalted butter, chopped
250 ml (9 fl oz/1 cup) rice malt syrup
½ teaspoon ground cinnamon
550 g (1 lb 4 oz/4 cups) toasted nut-free muesli
145 g (5 oz/1 cup) sesame seeds

STORAGE

The balls will keep in an airtight container in the fridge for up to 1 week.

1 Add the prunes to the mixer bowl, measuring cup in. Chop for 5 sec/speed 7, or until finely chopped. Scrape down the side of the bowl.

2 Add the butter to the mixer bowl, measuring cup in. Cook for 1 min/100°C/speed 2 or until melted.

3 Add the rice malt syrup, cinnamon and muesli to the mixer bowl, measuring cup in. Blend for 30 sec/speed 9, or until the mixture is well combined.

4 Using lightly damp hands, roll 1 tablespoon measures of the mixture into balls, then roll the balls in the sesame seeds to lightly coat. Transfer to an airtight container and chill.

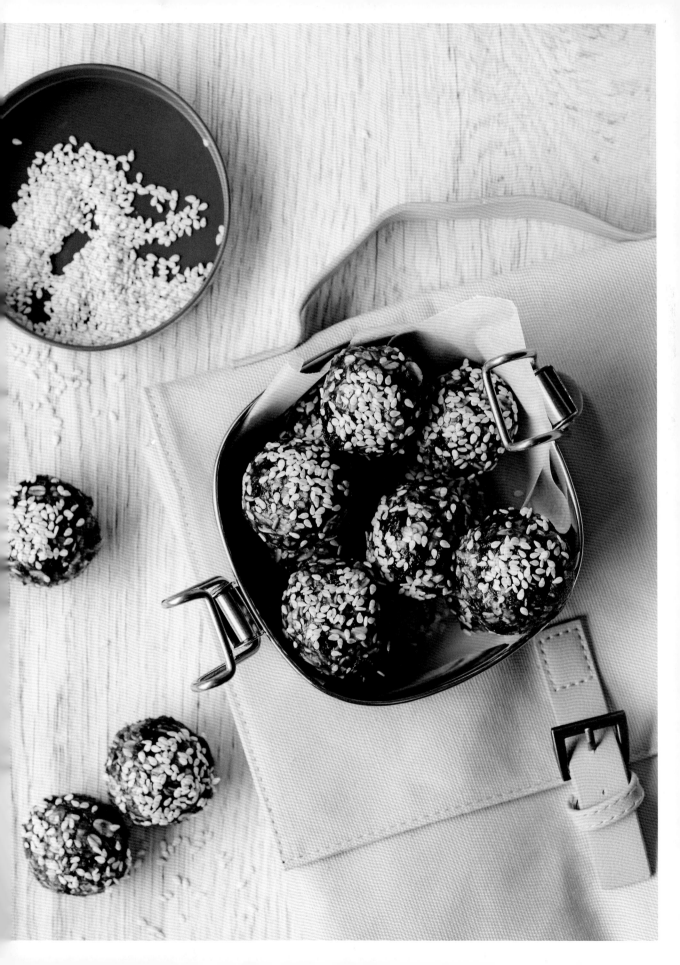

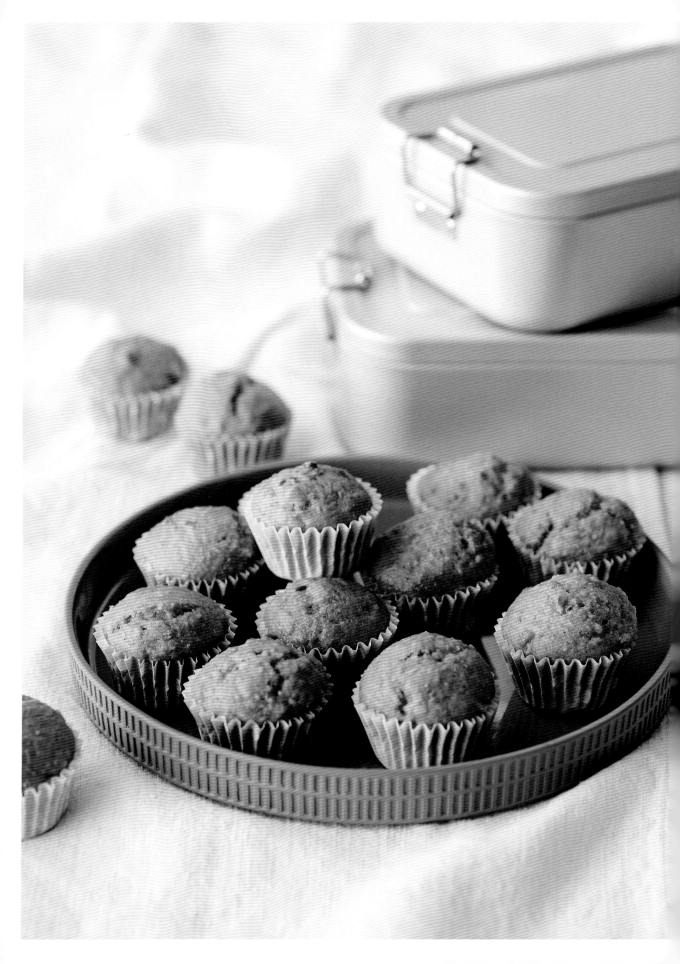

Mini apple banana muffins

makes 36
preparation 30 minutes, plus cooling time
cooking 20 minutes

1 medium green apple, skin on, cored,
  then cut into 3 cm (1¼ inch) pieces
2 ripe bananas, cut into 3
80 g (2¾ oz/½ cup) coconut sugar
2 eggs
125 ml (4 fl oz/½ cup) milk of choice
60 ml (2 fl oz/¼ cup) macadamia oil
½ teaspoon ground cinnamon
300 g (10½ oz/2 cups) self-raising wholemeal
  (whole-wheat) flour

STORAGE

The muffins will keep in an airtight container in a cool, dark place for up to 3 days, or in the fridge for up to 5 days. Separate into smaller portions in freezer-safe bags and freeze for up to 1 month.

1 Preheat the oven to 180°C (350°F)/160°C (315°F) fan-forced. Line 36 holes of two 24-hole, 2 tablespoon capacity mini muffin tins with paper cases.

2 Add the apple to the mixer bowl, measuring cup in. Grate for 3 sec/speed 6. Scrape down the side of the bowl.

3 Add the banana to the mixer bowl, measuring cup in. Blend for 3 sec/speed 7. Scrape down the side of the bowl.

4 Add the sugar, eggs, milk and oil to the mixer bowl, measuring cup in. Combine for 10 sec/reverse stir/speed 3. Scrape down the side of the bowl.

5 Add the cinnamon and flour to the mixer bowl, measuring cup in. Combine for 15 sec/reverse stir/speed 3.

6 Divide the mixture evenly among the prepared holes in the tins. Bake the muffins for 15–18 minutes, or until a skewer inserted in the centre comes out clean and the tops are golden. Cool in the tins for 3 minutes, then transfer to a wire rack to cool completely.

Strawberry cupcakes

makes 24
preparation 30 minutes, plus cooling time
cooking 25 minutes

110 g (3¾ oz/½ cup) white sugar
125 g (4½ oz) unsalted butter, at room temperature
300 g (10½ oz/2 cups) self-raising wholemeal
  (whole-wheat) flour
1 teaspoon pure vanilla extract
2 eggs
185 ml (6 fl oz/¾ cup) milk of choice
250 g (9 oz) strawberries, hulled and finely chopped
50 g (1¾ oz/¼ cup) raw (demerara) sugar

1 Preheat the oven to 180°C (350°F)/160°C (315°F) fan-forced. Line two
   12-hole, 80 ml (2½ fl oz/⅓ cup) capacity muffin tins with paper cases.

2 Add the white sugar to the mixer bowl, measuring cup in. Mill for
   10 sec/speed 10. Scrape down the side of the bowl.

3 Add the butter to the mixer bowl, measuring cup in. Mix for 10 sec/
   speed 4. Scrape down the side of the bowl.

4 Add the flour, vanilla, eggs and milk to the mixer bowl, measuring cup
   in. Blend for 10 sec/speed 5. Scrape down the side of the bowl. Blend
   for 10 sec/speed 5.

5 Divide half the mixture evenly among the holes in the prepared tins,
   sprinkle evenly with the strawberries, then spoon over the remaining
   mixture to cover. Sprinkle the tops with raw sugar.

6 Bake the cupcakes for 20–25 minutes or until a skewer inserted in
   the centre comes out clean, and the tops are golden. Cool in the tins
   for 5 minutes, then transfer to a wire rack to cool completely.

Banana pikelets

makes 48
preparation 20 minutes, plus cooling time
cooking 35 minutes

2 ripe bananas, cut into 3
300 g (10½ oz/2 cups) wholemeal
  (whole-wheat) self-raising flour
2 eggs
500 ml (17 fl oz/2 cups) milk of choice
2 teaspoons pure vanilla extract
olive oil cooking spray

STORAGE

The pikelets will keep in an
airtight container in a cool,
dark place for up to 3 days or
in the fridge for up to 5 days.
Separate into smaller portions
in freezer-safe bags and freeze
for up to 1 month.

1   Add the banana, flour, eggs, milk and vanilla to the mixer bowl,
    measuring cup in. Mix for 10 sec/speed 5 until smooth and combined.

2   Place a large non-stick frying pan over medium–high heat. Spray with
    oil to coat. Drop 1 tablespoon measures of the banana mixture into
    the pan, spreading to a 5 cm (2 inch) wide circle. Cook the pikelets,
    in batches, for 1–2 minutes or until bubbles appear on the surface and
    start to pop and are golden underneath. Flip, then cook for 1–2 minutes
    more or until golden. Transfer to a wire rack to cool.

Oaty apricot coconut bites

makes 30 pieces
preparation 30 minutes, plus cooling time
cooking 45 minutes

400 g (14 oz/4 cups) rolled (porridge) oats
180 g (6½ oz/2 cups) desiccated coconut
150 g (5½ oz/1 cup) wholemeal (whole-wheat) self-raising flour
310 g (11 oz/2 cups) dried apricots, cut in half
375 ml (13 fl oz/1½ cups) honey
250 g (9 oz) unsalted butter, chopped
80 g (2¾ oz/½ cup) coconut sugar

STORAGE

The bites will keep in an airtight container in a cool, dark place for up to 2 weeks. Separate into smaller portions in freezer-safe bags and freeze for up to 1 month.

1 Preheat the oven to 150°C (300°F)/130°C (250°F) fan-forced. Line the base and sides of a 35 x 25 x 2 cm (14 x 10 x ¾ inch) baking tray with baking paper.

2 Add the oats to the mixer bowl, measuring cup in. Mill for 10 sec/speed 9. Scrape down the side of the bowl. Mill for 10 sec/speed 9. Transfer the mixture to a large heatproof bowl. Add the desiccated coconut and flour and stir to combine. Clean the mixer bowl.

3 Add the apricots to the mixer bowl, measuring cup in. Chop for 20 sec/speed 7. Scrape down the side of the bowl.

4 Add the remaining ingredients to the mixer bowl, measuring cup in. Cook for 3 min/100°C/speed 2 until the butter melts and the sugar has dissolved. Transfer to the oat mixture in the bowl and stir to combine.

5 Spoon the apricot mixture into the prepared tray, pressing it down firmly and evenly. Bake for 35–40 minutes or until golden and firm. Cool completely in the tray. Remove and cut into 30 pieces.

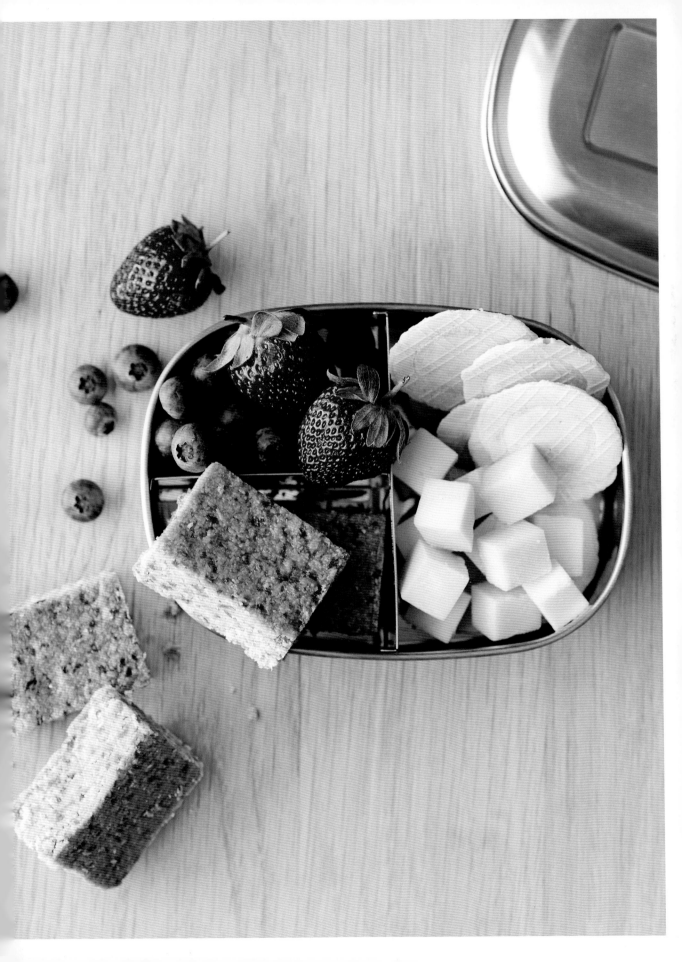

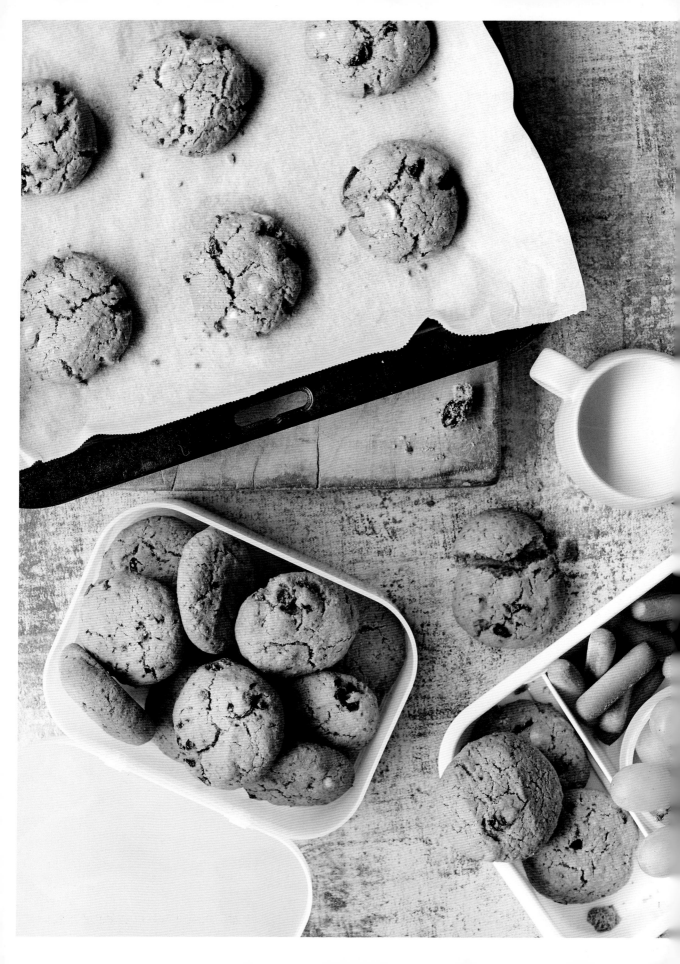

Cranberry and white choc chip cookies

makes 28
preparation 30 minutes, plus cooling time
cooking 30 minutes

125 g (4½ oz) unsalted butter, at room temperature
120 g (4¼ oz/¾ cup) coconut sugar
1 egg
2 teaspoons pure vanilla extract
300 g (10½ oz/2 cups) wholemeal (whole-wheat)
  self-raising flour
75 g (2½ oz/½ cup) reduced-sugar dried
  cranberries
85 g (3 oz/½ cup) white chocolate baking chips

STORAGE

The cookies will keep in an airtight container in a cool, dark place for up to 1 week.

1 Preheat the oven to 160°C (315°F)/140°C (275°F) fan-forced. Line four large baking trays with baking paper.

2 Add the butter, sugar, egg and vanilla to the mixer bowl, measuring cup in. Mix for 2 min/speed 3. Scrape down the side of the bowl.

3 Add the flour, dried cranberries and chocolate chips to the mixer bowl, measuring cup in. Mix for 2 min/speed 3. Scrape down the side of the bowl.

4 Roll 1 tablespoon measures of the mixture into balls. Place on the prepared trays and flatten them slightly. Bake two trays of cookies at a time, swapping them around on the shelves halfway through baking, for 15 minutes each or until light golden. Cool the cookies on the trays.

index

Published in 2020 by Murdoch Books, an imprint of Allen & Unwin

Murdoch Books Australia
83 Alexander Street,
Crows Nest NSW 2065
Phone: +61 (0) 2 8425 0100
murdochbooks.com.au
info@murdochbooks.com.au

Murdoch Books UK
Ormond House, 26–27 Boswell Street
London WC1N 3JZ
Phone: +44 (0) 20 8785 5995
murdochbooks.co.uk
info@murdochbooks.co.uk

For corporate orders and custom publishing, contact our business
development team at salesenquiries@murdochbooks.com.au

Publisher: Jane Morrow
Editorial Manager: Virginia Birch
Design Manager: Vivien Valk
Concept and cover design: Madeleine Kane
Designer: Susanne Geppert
Editor: Ariana Klepac
Photographer: Cath Muscat
Stylist: Bhavani Konings
Home Economist: Theressa Klein/Sarah Mayoh
Production Director: Lou Playfair

ISBN 978 1 76052 524 8 Australia
ISBN 978 1 91163 255 9 UK

A catalogue record for this
book is available from the
National Library of Australia

A catalogue record for this book is available from the British Library

Colour reproduction by Splitting Image Colour Studio Pty Ltd, Clayton, Victoria
Printed by C & C Offset Printing Co. Ltd., China

TABLESPOON MEASURES: We have used 20 ml (4 teaspoon) tablespoon measures. If you are using a 15 ml (3 teaspoon)
tablespoon add an extra teaspoon of the ingredient for each tablespoon specified.

**DISCLAIMER: The purchaser of this book understands that the operating information contained within is not intended
to replace the thermo appliance instructions supplied by the manufacturer. The author and publisher claim no
responsibility to any person or entity for any liability, loss, damage or injury caused or alleged to be caused directly
or indirectly as a result of the use, application or interpretation of the material in this book. It is understood that you
will carefully follow the safety instructions supplied by the manufacturer before operating your thermo appliance.**

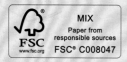

The paper in this book is FSC® certified.
FSC® promotes environmentally responsible,
socially beneficial and economically viable
management of the world's forests.

**ACKNOWLEDGEMENT
OF COUNTRY**
**The author acknowledges
the traditional owners of the
Country that this cookbook
was created on, the Gadigal
people of the Eora nation, and
recognises their continuing
connection to land, waters
and culture. The author pays
her respects to Elders past,
present and emerging.**